CHANGE OF LIFE

Marie-Louise von Franz, Honorary Patron

**Studies in Jungian Psychology
by Jungian Analysts**

Daryl Sharp, General Editor

CHANGE OF LIFE

A Psychological Study
of
Dreams and the Menopause

ANN MANKOWITZ

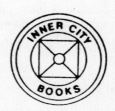

INNER CITY BOOKS

To Julia and her daughters

Canadian Cataloguing in Publication Data

Mankowitz, Ann
    Change of life

(Studies in Jungian psychology by Jungian analysts; 16)

Bibliography: p.
Includes index.

ISBN 0-919123-15-5

1. Menopause—Psychological aspects. 2. Jung, C. G.
(Carl Gustav), 1875-1961. I. Title. II. Series.

RG186.M36 1984   618.1′75   C84-098309-3

INNER CITY BOOKS
Box 1271, Station Q, Toronto, Canada M4T 2P4
Telephone (416) 927-0355

Honorary Patron: Marie-Louise von Franz.
Publisher and General Editor: Daryl Sharp.
Editorial Board: Fraser Boa, Daryl Sharp, Marion Woodman.

INNER CITY BOOKS was founded in 1980 to promote the
understanding and practical application of the work of C.G. Jung.

Cover: The Passage of Time—from an old copy of the *Saturday
Evening Post* (artist unknown).

Glossary and Index by Daryl Sharp.

Printed and bound in Canada by Webcom Limited

CONTENTS

See final pages for descriptions of other INNER CITY BOOKS

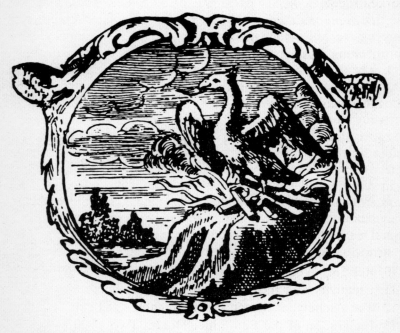

The mythological phoenix, symbol of rebirth (see pages 72-75).
(Boschius, *Symbolographia,* 1702)

Introduction

This book is about a woman I call Rachel, and the extraordinary dreams she had in the course of her analysis with me. It is also about the menopause, because at the time of her analysis Rachel was going through "the change of life." As we worked together on her dreams I found myself waking up for the first time to the special significance of the menopause, not only for Rachel herself, but also for me and for other women approaching or experiencing this crucial period in their lives.

I was practicing as a Jungian analyst in Dublin when Rachel appeared on the scene. She was in analysis with me altogether for nearly three years. When she first came she was fifty-one and had just had her final menstruation. Aware as she was of being in a crisis of mid-life, with the role changes and adjustments to aging which this implied, she nevertheless referred only rarely in any direct way to the menopause, and I, in common with many others (notably, as I discovered later, women like myself approaching menopause), also evaded conscious awareness of the menopause as a specific psychosomatic event of middle age.

Rachel's approach to psychotherapy was an important factor in her experience ultimately becoming the basis of my research into the menopause. She came into analysis in the first place not because she was suffering from depression or any disturbing "menopausal" symptoms. She was a healthy and well-adjusted woman with a grown-up family, a good marriage and work which interested her. Yet she had a feeling of emptiness, she felt her femininity was threatened and her life seemed lacking in direction. Because she had heard that Jungians believe in the "second half of life," the postbiological phase, as a time for personal integration and self-discovery, she hoped that a Jungian analysis would help her to find meaning at this critical stage of her life. She did not enter analysis wanting the sort of help that tranquilizes; she wished to confront the realities of her own experience in the fullest,

7

most conscious way. She chose analysis as she had in the past chosen natural childbirth—because she was the sort of person who wanted to understand every experience with as much of herself as possible.

Both Rachel and her husband were English and had lived most of their lives in England, until three years previously when they moved to Ireland for reasons connected with his work. Their three grown-up children remained in England: two sons of twenty-nine and twenty-six, the older married with a baby girl of two; and a daughter of nineteen who was at university and had been away from home for a year, although she spent some part of her holidays with her parents.

After thirty years of marriage and family life, Rachel and her husband Phil were living alone together in a small house in the country just outside Dublin. Phil was a professor of architecture, and had written books on the subject. He was a year older than Rachel. Their marriage had been fairly stormy but it had lasted. Family life was important to both, and they were, at this stage, usually good companions, with love and respect for each other and the children. They still enjoyed each other sexually, though rather less frequently than before in their early and mid-forties. Rachel, after acquiring a degree in social science, had not worked until her youngest child went to school. She then trained and worked as a marital therapist for eight years in England, and was working in Dublin as a marriage counselor when she came to me. Phil's parents and Rachel's father had all died several years before. Her mother died about a year before she started analysis. Rachel herself was a trim, attractive woman, who obviously took good care of herself and her appearance.

The key position of one woman's dreams and dream-work in this study of the menopause derives from the basic principles of C.G. Jung's analytical psychology. Most relevant is Jung's belief that dreams have an important guiding and compensatory function, particularly helpful in the critical passages of life:

The unconscious content [of dreams] contrasts strikingly with the conscious material, particularly when the conscious attitude tends too exclusively in a direction that would threaten the vital needs of the individual.... Vivid dreams with a strongly contrasting but purposive content will appear as an expression of the self-regulation of the psyche...just as the body reacts purposively to injuries or infections.[1]

In other words, work on a vivid dream, one remembered in detail, reveals and encourages the natural inclination of the psyche toward wholeness in a time of crisis. Analytic work on dreams can thus not only facilitate self-discovery and the individual therapeutic process, which is its chief function, but may also be used as data for more general research into the crisis through which the dreamer is passing.

In Rachel's case, dreams gave us access to her unconscious in the critical period of the menopause. The dream imagery yielded up its meaning not only because of its personal associations for Rachel, but also because of the *archetypal* nature of its symbolism. Archetypal images are those universal symbols that appear in cultures all over the world and in every age—in myths, religious rites, folklore, works of art and literature—and they arise unbidden in dreams.

In any depth analysis, the continuing work of association, amplification and interpretation of imagery, based on established psychoanalytic and Jungian theory, is focused upon spontaneous products of the unconscious, of which the dream is the most spontaneous and the least censored by reason and thought. As Joseph Campbell writes:

The human kingdom, beneath the floor of the comparatively neat little dwelling that we call our consciousness, goes down into unsuspected Aladdin caves. There not only jewels but also dangerous jinn abide: the inconvenient or resisted psychological powers that we have not thought or dared to integrate into our lives....

Psychoanalysis, the modern science of reading dreams, has taught us to take heed of these unsubstantial images. *Also it has found a way to let them do their work.* The dangerous crises of self-development are permitted to come to pass under the protecting eye of an experienced initiate in the lore and language of dreams.[2]

The first of Rachel's three so-called big dreams (those of particular significance) occurred about half way through her analysis, when she had encountered many of the resistances which are part of the analytic relationship and, without being aware of it, was well into the process of psychic adjustment to her physiological changes. At crucial times of development, the conscious mind takes a long time to catch up with and integrate both the bodily changes and the unconscious adjustments of the psyche. It often takes a significant dream to do it, and this seems particularly true during the change of life.

It was not until the session in which Rachel first told the dream that I started to think more deeply about the menopause and its neglected significance in the lives of my patients and myself. The dream began like this:

> I am walking round the house in the country, our family home where we all lived when my children were younger. It's burnt out, destroyed by fire, a blackened empty shell. Parts of it look like dead petrified trees, some of it twisted like flames solidified. I am alone . . . utterly desolate. It's me, my insides, my womb . . . but not just that . . . my past life, my children . . . the whole way of life ended forever . . . but round at the back of the house there is new grass growing, and that gives me hope.

Her instant intuition, her strong feeling in the telling and the vivid imagery of this initial fragment struck chords in me, and as the dream-work went on I started asking myself questions:

What is the menopause? Is it really an important and crucial event? If so, to whom? To the individual women who experience it? To society, the collective? If it is a significant stage of life, why is it so neglected? Why do women themselves avoid talking about it, deny knowledge of it? What is the stereotype of the menopausal woman? Is it changing? Is the menopause a time of loss or a time of liberation? Or both?

The purpose of this book is to offer some answers to these broader questions, while maintaining a psychological focus on one menopausal woman's dreams and experience.

PART I

PRELIMINARY CONSIDERATIONS

1

What is the Menopause?

Initial Research

As the work on Rachel's first dream progressed, I became increasingly more aware and more curious about the menopause, reading and talking about it whenever the opportunity arose. Before looking in detail at Rachel's dreams and the course of her analysis I want to present some of my initial findings.

Neither reading nor talking were as simple as expected; the literature was sparse, and most women seemed unwilling even to think about the menopause. It became clear that the first reaction to the very idea was an evasive or denying one. While I was in Dublin, I was surprised to find that those most interested in the subject were *young* people, of both sexes, who had been affected by their mothers' menopause. One young man told me that his mother's "change" came when he was fourteen, and she did indeed change toward him—from an affectionate and indulgent parent to a moody and rejecting one. Unable to understand what was happening, he felt confused, miserable and guilty. Naturally he felt that the whole subject needed to be brought into the open.

But the middle-aged did not share his enthusiasm and the women showed markedly ambivalent attitudes. They did not want to acknowledge the menopause, or its imminence and inevitability for *them;* at the same time, in spite of themselves, they were desperately anxious to know more and to find out what *I* knew and would share with them. Psychologist Abraham Maslow called this syndrome "the need to know and the fear of knowing."[3]

When later (some months after the end of Rachel's analysis) I moved into rural Ireland in County Cork, I found very much the same ambivalence. Returning at frequent intervals to my home-base in London, I talked to friends, relations and colleagues there about the menopause; and subsequently in my travels in the United States, I pursued the subject in New York, Texas, New Mexico and California, and found the same "fear of knowing" and the same "need to know." Gradually, however, inspired by the themes which had emerged from the work on Rachel's dreams, as I listened to menopausal women in all these places I discovered both variations in attitude, arising from different socio-cultural backgrounds, and also the universality of experience which was shared by all women.

During the time I was talking to individuals and groups in Europe and America, I was also reading everything I could about the menopause. But it was not easy to find.

In the literature of depth psychology and anthropology there was very little about the menopause. Of the Freudian psychoanalysts, Helene Deutsch had written the most extensively and sensitively on the subject.[4] Among Jungian writers, there was no direct reference to the menopause, but their historical and mythological material on the goddess-centered religions, fertility cults and moon symbolism threw much light on the imagery of Rachel's dreams,[5] as did the work of religious historian Mircea Eliade and mythographer Joseph Campbell.[6] Anthropologist J.G. Frazer wrote a good deal about the taboos of menstruation,[7] and Margaret Mead examined the role of postmenopausal women in certain primitive cultures,[8] but it seemed clear that the menopause was and is virtually a non-event in all societies.

In the years between 1973 and 1977, there seems to have been very little research on the menopause, most of it in the United States, though some in Britain and Europe. I found only twenty or so articles from almost as many different specialist journals covering almost as many different aspects of the menopause.

The fewest contributions were from general psychiatry; these dealt mostly with the nursing of affective disorders and the administration of drugs and hormones. The most numerous contributions were from the journals of geriatric and developmental psychology, with articles about self-image, family relationships and separation crises, all in relation to aging. In the journals of gynecology, psychosomatic medicine and medical education, the subjects were hormone replacement and symptoms and management of the menopause. In journals of clinical and social psychology, there were articles on mid-age crisis, psychosexual problems and changing roles in society.

In spite of the sparseness of the material, it seemed there were many ways of looking at the menopause. It could be seen as a deficiency disease, a neurosis, a social problem or as a symptom of aging. Few of the writers treated it with the generally positive consideration given to other major developmental changes in life.

During my initial research, I came across three books about the menopause written by women. The first was by an English journalist. It was well researched and full of factual information, but was basically propaganda for hormone replacement therapy, which it was claimed would impart everlasting youthful vigor and, if desired, a lifelong menstrual cycle. Hence the title, *No Change*.[9]

The second book was called *Menstruation and Menopause*, a pioneering and comprehensive study by a New York psychologist,[10] perhaps the first ever on the subject written out of a woman's own experience.

The third book, *Menopause: A Positive Approach*, was by an American feminist journalist.[11] Against hormone replacement and in favor of natural health foods and self-help medicine, this author's "positive" approach nevertheless contained a denial of change, particularly sexual change. She stridently maintained that sex is better when you're older.

A fourth book, though not specifically about the menopause, is worth mentioning. *The Wise Wound* was written by a man and a woman (both professional writers), and offered an original viewpoint on the menstrual cycle.[12] With abundant illustration from myth and folklore, the writers attempted to redress the balance between the accepted ideas about menstruation and the actual function of ovulation, and to approach the menstrual function in a new and genuinely positive way for women.

There also emerged around this time a type of literature from the women's movements with a sexual-political orientation different from that of such disparate feminist writers as Simone de Beauvoir, Betty Friedan, Kate Millett and Germaine Greer. Instead of regarding female biology as an unfair handicap, which has to be ignored or overcome in order to get an equal share of rights in a man's world, this new generation from Britain and the United States seemed more inclined to reassess and revalue female human nature, in both its physical and psychological aspects, and to aim for a world more in accordance with the feminine principle than hitherto male-dominated society had allowed.[13] Apart from some extreme female chauvinism, this new emphasis struck me as particularly relevant to the feminine experience I was examining.

More recent material on the subject tends to focus on the physiological changes women may expect at the menopause, and even though some writers also consider the social and psychological factors, they do not extend their attention to the possible significance of dreams.

Defining the Change

Here are some of the definitions and descriptions of the menopause I came upon in the course of my reading:

> *Menopause (Climacteric).* A term that implies the final cessation of menstruation and therefore the end of a woman's reproductive life. (*Encyclopedia Brittanica,* 1970)

> Evolution has set another brake on female enterprise and energy, coming into operation in mid-life in the form of the *menopause.* More correctly the whole process of de-generation starting with the atrophy and shut down of the ovaries and continuing through to old age is known as the *climacteric.* The

menopause strictly means only "final menstruation." (Wendy Cooper, *No Change*)

The physical and emotional transition from middle to old age is called the *climacteric.* Men and women experience many identical changes during this fifteen-year period, but *menopause,* which occurs during *climacteric,* is unique to females. After twelve consecutive months of no menstruation, fertility has ended and menopause is a fact of life. (Paula Weideger, *Menstruation and Menopause*)

The menopause (also called the climacteric or change of life) marks the end of the reproductive part of a woman's life. Its chief outward sign is the cessation of the monthly flow of menstrual blood. (Diagram Group, *Woman's Body: An Owner's Manual*)

Menopause is defined as the point of cessation of menstruation. It is brought on by the gradual decline in estrogen level production by the ovaries over several years, to the point where menstrual bleeding actually ceases. The symptoms may include a gradual decrease in menstrual flow, a decrease in predictability of the cycle, or, in a few women, an abrupt cessation of menstruation. For most women the onset of menopause occurs between the ages of forty-five and fifty, but it can begin earlier or later. When a woman has had no period for twelve months she is considered to be "through menopause." The term climacteric refers to the whole process of transition in ovarian and hormonal function while the term menopause refers to the cessation of menstruation. (Kathie Smallwood and Dorothy Van Dyck, "Menopause Counseling")

We see here an interesting variety of views. The menopause and the climacteric are the same for the *Encyclopedia* and the *Owner's Manual.* Cooper, Weideger and Smallwood make a distinction between them. Only the *Owner's Manual* (the most recent of the books quoted) mentions the term "change of life." This common usage has more impact than the scientific "menopause," which suggests that though menstruation has ceased, it might at some future time start up again. The everyday term "change of life" shows a recognition (whether conscious or unconscious) that the change is a fundamental and permanent one. Most significantly, both Cooper and the study by Smallwood and Van Dyck do not mention in their definitions the ending of reproductivity; the cessation of menstruation seems for them to be unconnected with fertility.

The above descriptions also show some disagreement over the use of the words "menopause" and "climacteric." In this book I have not employed the term "climacteric," partly because it is used in relation to men as well as women and this is a study of women, and partly because I have stretched the more generally used "menopause" and "change of life" to cover the variable span of time, from five to ten years, during which a woman gradually ceases to menstruate, finally ceases to be fertile and subsequently comes to assimilate into her experience of herself the changes in her bodily and emotional life. Women who have had hysterectomies, and therefore "false" menopauses, also experience a "natural" menopause, both through the changes in their ovarian hormones, and through their life-experience at that time. I acknowledge that after menstruation has ceased for one year, a woman may be said to be "postmenopausal." Nevertheless, my own usage of the term "menopause" to cover the psychological assimilation of all physical changes, includes also the pre- and post-menopausal periods.

In spite of all the shades of difference in definition, can the menopause as a physiological event be described with precision? In the session after telling her first dream, Rachel asked: "What is actually happening inside my body? In one way, I know, but the objective facts I don't know much about."

Rachel was not the only one to be vague about the physiological processes taking place in a woman's body at this time. Even the medical authorities themselves do not agree about the exact mechanisms of either the menstrual cycle or the menopause. As the authors of *The Wise Wound* point out:

It is only since 1930 that the uncertainties about whether womb-lining was shed and when in the cycle the egg was released were more or less resolved. The changes that occur in the womb-lining were not fully described until 1950 ... [just as] it was not until 1966 that there was any reliable account of what happened in people's physiology when they made love.[14]

What Rachel knew from her own experience is described in a more general way by Bernice Neugarten:

In some women the menstrual cycle ceases very abruptly, but more often its disappearance is gradual. A period or two is skipped, then menstruation recurs more or less normally from one to several times, then there is again a period of amenorrhea which may last several months, and so on until complete cessation. This "dodging period" of the menopause may go on for a year or two, sometimes longer. The amount and duration of the menstrual flow may be normal until the very end, but frequently there is a gradual diminution of both.

The loss of the childbearing function is brought about by progressive and irreversible changes which occur in the ovaries as a result of that mysterious process called aging. While aging itself is by no means understood, it is nevertheless well established that the human ovary has a functional life of about 35 years. Over this period of time the ability of the ova to mature gradually diminishes, and finally ovulation stops. The production of ovarian hormones decreases, and then falls below the level capable of producing bleeding from the walls of the uterus.

The underlying hormonal activities are extraordinarily complex.... Certain hormones produced by the pituitary ... rise to high levels, affecting the vasomotor system, which in turn produces certain physiological symptoms, primarily the so-called "hot flash" or "hot flush" ... regarded as the most characteristic symptom of the menopause.[15]

Dr. John Studd is a consultant gynecologist at King's College Hospital, London, and runs one of the few menopause clinics in England. Here is part of his account of the physiological changes that occur at the menopause:

The ovary contains the maximum number of öocytes (egg-cells) during the fifth month of foetal life. Thereafter the numbers decline and only one million are present at birth and as few as twenty-five thousand remain at the menopause, at which time the ovary fails to ovulate and to produce hormones. Even before the periods cease, plasma levels of oestrone, oestradiol, progesterone and testosterone fall and at the same time there is an increase in the pituitary gonadotrophins, follicle-stimulating hormone (FSH) and luteinizing hormone (LH).

The senescent ovary shrinks and the vulva, vagina, uterus, Fallopian tubes, pelvic ligaments and breasts all take part in a general tissue atrophy. The skin loses collagen and becomes more dry and inelastic, and the bladder mucosa and periurethral supporting vascular tissues involute.... After several years osteoporosis may be evident.... At the same time women lose their relative immunity to coronary thrombosis....

Symptomatology. With the exception of the characteristic vasomotor symptoms, flushes and sweats, the symptoms of the climacteric are common to many other emotional, domestic, cosmetic and skeletal changes of aging.... Atrophic vaginitis may produce dyspareunia and post-menopausal bleeding as well as more subtle complaints of a dry vagina during intercourse and a fall in libido.[16]

This was the most comprehensive account I found of the physiological changes. It embraces the fascinating information about the presence of egg cells in the female baby and the course of their decline; something of the complex processes of the hormonal system; and, with a greater impact on the lay imagination, the stark facts of bodily decay. Although I find Studd's tone negative and pessimistic, at least he takes the menopausal changes seriously. While believing that some of the physical suffering of women at menopause can be alleviated by hormone replacement, he feels many of their problems are due not to the menopause itself, but simply to aging and other stresses at this time of life:

Behavioural changes such as insomnia, fatigue, depression, irritability and forgetfulness are common at this age. If these are of recent onset, they may respond to oestrogen therapy, but this will clearly have no effect on the despair produced by the realisation of an unfulfilled life brought into focus by departing children, troublesome aged parents and a husband preoccupied with other things.[17]

These aspects of mid-life—the marital, familial and social—can be as much a part of the total experience of the menopausal woman as the flushes and the hormones, but not necessarily so. Many women suffer neither the physical nor the psychological symptoms.

Perhaps the most fateful part of the physio-socio-psychodrama of female human life is the earliest, when the tiny female is waiting in the wings and not yet on stage: when she is still in her mother's womb and already fully equipped herself with womb, ovaries and her full complement of around a million egg cells. She is clearly designed to be a reproductive being.

At puberty, usually around a girl's early teens, there is increased activity in the glands producing female hormones, and she starts to menstruate, the sign that before long she will be into her fertile years and will be capable, with the cooperation of a male partner, of producing offspring.

In the thirty-five or forty years between menarche (the first menstrual period) and menopause, she experiences constant reminders of the reproductive nature of her physiology. Even if she has no children, her body demonstrates every month that her womb is in a state of readiness to have them. If she has children, she experiences the indelible imprint upon her whole natural system of the pregnancies, the births and subsequent prolonged nurturing of these children.

Then, around the mid to late forties, menopause starts and reverses the process of puberty, so that the glands producing female sex hormones decrease their activity. By the time a woman is in her early fifties, menstruation has ceased and she is no longer fertile.

As we have seen, the menopausal syndrome has two main physiological components: the loss of reproductivity, just mentioned, and also the loss of ovarian hormones. This latter loss affects her sexually, in the following way. Although it seems she can be as sexually desirous, and as sexually active, as before—and perhaps even more so with the end of menstruation and the removal of pregnancy fear—yet the decrease in the hormone estrogen has the effect of shrinking and drying the internal and external sex organs, and skin and tissues share a general thinning process. In other words, the body ages and loses, at varying rates, its physical attractions and its readiness for sexual intercourse.

At this point in the drama our heroine is in a sad plight, faced with a triple renunciation of youth, fertility and sexual power, and apparently without any hope of rescue.

2

The Neglected Crisis

Rites of Passage

Why is the menopause, ostensibly a momentous event in the life of the individual woman, so neglected by society, by history, by mythology and by religion? Why, for instance, are there no rites of passage recorded *anywhere* to mark out the menopause, as there are for other crucial events such as birth, puberty, marriage, childbirth and death?

The function of a rite of passage is to give significance to a crucial change in the life of the individual, to give one the support of society during this change and to attempt by means of the ritual to bring down the blessing of the gods at this time of danger both to the individual and to society. Rites of passage usually take place in three parts: first, the stage of isolation, withdrawal of the individual from society and into close contact with, and dependence upon, nature; second, the ordeal of severance, an event sometimes painful, involving physical or symbolic renunciation and confrontation with loss and death; and third, a ceremony of rebirth and renewal—the return of a changed being into society and the world.[18]

It can be seen that the pattern of these religious rites (which is a universal one) reflects the inner pattern of individual experience in times of fundamental change. As Joseph Campbell writes:

> A great number of the ritual trials and images correspond to those that appear automatically in dreams the moment the psychoanalyzed patient begins to abandon his infantile fixations and to progress into the future. . . .
>
> It has always been the prime function of mythology and rite to supply the symbols that carry the human spirit forward, in counteraction to those other constant human fantasies that tend to tie it back.[19]

It is the acting out of these rites that makes the changes

20

bearable and valuable, and gives them a meaning shared by society and society's gods. The menopause, however, though specifically called *the change of life,* never seems to have had the benefit of this sanction. Why not? Let us consider some facts which may provide a partial answer.

In the Roman Empire, the life expectancy of a woman was twenty-five years; in the fifteenth century it was thirty years; by Victorian times it had only risen to forty-five years; and even at the beginning of this century it was only fifty years.[20] Although these are of course average figures, brought down by the high rate of infant mortality, it does seem as if few women lived much beyond the menopause. There is some evidence that in earlier times the menopause occurred around the mid-forties rather than the fifties, but even so, fewer women would have experienced any length of postmenopausal life compared to those who do today.

There are other reasons for neglect in the past besides the generally shorter life span. One is suggested by Robert Richardson:

> We must ask why an event of such significance to the individual woman passed almost without notice sociologically, anthropologically and medically. And the answer thrown back from the silent past is that the menopause was a negative event of no importance in the life of the community. So when a woman's usefulness was seen to be ended, she ceased to be a woman.[21]

This is a clear statement of a particularly patriarchal attitude: When a woman can no longer bear children, she is no longer of use. This attitude still persists overtly in many parts of the world, and probably unconsciously in many men and women everywhere, and it certainly accounts for much of the neglect of the menopause. But the belief that she loses her womanhood reflects less conscious attitudes of patriarchal society, which may have more bearing on the present day. These concern the sexual power the nubile woman has traditionally possessed, reflected in the taboos of menstruation.

The human menstrual cycle is entirely different from the

animal oestrus, although until fairly recently they were thought to be equivalent. In fact, there is still a great deal of mystery surrounding the origin and purpose of menstruation. According to the authors of *The Wise Wound:*

> *It is received opinion in zoological science that the development of the menstrual cycle was responsible for the evolution of primate and eventually human societies....*
>
> Most of the animals, right upwards in the evolutionary series through the mammals, have specific breeding-times and seasons, and these are the only times that they are inspired with sexual energy to beget offspring. At other times animals are not interested in mating. This is because the majority of the mammals have an *oestrus* cycle, and they come "on heat" at specific times.
>
> The menstrual cycle is continuous—unlike the oestrus cycle of many animals, which have longish resting-phases with no discernible ovarian activity at all. Another difference is that in most *oestrus* cycles a little blood is shed at the *ovulation* and this is a powerful mating-signal. In the menstrual cycle, the blood is shed with the womb-wall.... It is as though the mating-signal of genital blood has been wrenched from its former position at ovulation, to a new position at menstruation, when it is very unlikely that ovulation can occur, or offspring can be conceived. It is as though what this evolutionary step meant was that sex was now to be used for something other than reproduction, since sexual libido was also wrenched from its former exclusive attachment to the ripening of the egg, and spread over most of the cycle, with another concentration of sexual interest at or around menstruation. Yet how, ask the evolutionists, can this be of benefit to the species, since menstruation is a "safe" period, and offspring cannot usually result at this time?[22]

So the menstrual cycle not only separates sexuality from reproduction, but also appears to increase sexual attraction at just that time in the cycle when fertility is at its lowest (i.e., menstruation time) which would seem to go against the interests of the species. To counteract this attraction, the taboo of menstruation arose. It is only fair to say that there are many opinions about the reasons for the menstrual taboo, yet it is generally agreed that, as in the case of the incest taboo (which may be associated with it), so strict a proscription as a taboo only arises where desire for the tabooed object is very strong indeed.

Whatever its origins, it was this taboo which reflected and increased the awesome power of nubile women, and made them at their time of menstruation both sacred and deadly. It was the loss of this power at menopause which deprived women of their status in later life. Writes Paula Weideger:

> In our culture a woman is sexually desirable only as long as her sexuality can also inspire fear. Once she no longer menstruates, she is assumed to have lost her sexuality. . . . Our cultural inheritance has dictated that woman is valued and valuable only as long as she can reproduce.[23]

This describes, not a conscious attitude, but a cultural inheritance which embodies the age-old universal image of the magical power of the fertile woman. As different as our modern rational notions of fertility are, we are still unconsciously influenced by archaic beliefs and taboos. Modern men may or may not be aware of fear, or modern women of magical power, but it is these elements, as well as the obvious social necessity for females to carry on the race, that give the nubile woman her special value in society.

History tells us that, with some exceptions, both the matriarchal, goddess-centered cultures, and the patriarchal, male-dominated ones have proved equally remiss in giving a position of dignity and worth to the postfertile woman; the first because of the worship of female fertility power, and the second because of the repression of female power in general.

The Older Woman in Society

What is or has been the role, if any, of the postmenopausal woman in society?

Elaine Morgan's research into prehistoric times led her to the idea of the grandmothers as oral educators and storytellers of the tribe; indeed, she sees this as their evolutionary raison d'être:

One of the most vital factors in human evolutionary success was the power to accumulate knowledge, to profit not only from personal experience but from the experience of others, even of others long dead. Before the invention of writing this was made possible only by the long life and memory of older members of the tribe.... The only way of accounting for the evolutionary emergence of the menopause in women is by the assumption that the tribe as a whole, and not merely the individual, derived some benefit from the presence of those females who, although sterile, lived to a ripe and healthy old age. In some way or other, and in a way that applied to other species that we know of, grannies were good for them.[24]

In 1949, Margaret Mead described the situation in Bali:

The post-menopausal woman and the virgin girl work together at ceremonies from which women of childbearing age are debarred. Where modesty of speech and action is enjoined on women, such behaviour may no longer be asked of older women who may use obscene language as freely or more freely than any man.[25]

According to Paula Weideger, in China before the revolution the postmenopausal woman had a secure and coveted position; for the first time in her life she could shake off male domination, and, with the approval of society, even assume domination over males.[26]

American sociologist Pauline Bart, who studied anthropological accounts of the status of women in a great number of cultures, discovered that in spite of an enormous variation in concepts of feminity, the feminine role assumed in the fertile years of a woman's life was in all cultures reversed after menopause.[27] The examples from Bali and China bear this out, and demonstrate particularly a reversal of sex-role.

The idea of the older woman losing her femininity with her fertility and joining the men, so to speak, may penetrate to inner feelings as well as to social practices. Vieda Skultans made a study of rural Welsh women in 1970 and found several at the menopause who felt they were changing structurally and anatomically into men. One said, "Women turn into men inside," and another reported that she felt "a turning and tightening of the thigh muscles."[28]

Witchcraft was probably one way in which the old goddess religions survived after being driven underground. Historically witches have been of all ages and both sexes, but the concept of the witch that has come down to us in folklore and fairytale is that of a malicious and ugly old hag. There is a connection here with the image of the menopausal woman. "Many of the witches killed were old women since 'the devil walks in a dry place.'"[29] So-called witch ointment, used by women in the menopause, was probably composed mainly of menstrual blood, and the only time when a woman could not be a witch was when she was bearing a child.[30]

We often think of the wise women, healers and midwives of the past, as well as the priestesses, sybils and oracles of classical times, as having been older women. History tells us that although there may be some truth in this (Esther Harding refers to the "ancient priestesses" of the moon goddess),[31] in many cases these roles were filled by younger women, sometimes dedicated to these vocations in early youth.

In fact the evidence of the part played by the postfertile woman in the life of her society is sparse and often conjectural. General neglect and masculine bias can be partly blamed for this, but we know from the statistics that this is due also to the shortness of life in the past, which meant that few women lived for very long once they had passed the menopause.

Nowadays, however, an enormous number of women live for a long span after they have ceased to be reproductive:

In the U.S. just over 20% of the female population is over 55. Life expectancy for the average American woman is 76. With the menopause occurring at around 50 these women may well have a third of their lives to come. Their life situation is very different from that at the turn of the century, when life expectancy was 50 years and the menopause occurred in the mid or late forties.[32]

The contemporary social situation demands a different continuity and a different psychological response from that of the past. No longer can society afford to ignore its menopausal and postmenopausal women, constituting as they do such a sizable proportion of the total population. Equally important, women themselves need to emerge from their historic doldrums and develop positive attitudes in response to the fact that modern technology has bestowed upon them an average twenty-five years of life after the menopause.

In spite of, or perhaps because of, the decrease in birth rate and the increase in the aging population, affluent Western consumer societies have until very recently had little use for their old people, little respect for their potential wisdom and experience; on the contrary, giving value only to youth and economic productivity, they have tended to regard their old as a dangerous burden.

The position of women in general in these societies has altered considerably in recent times. Widespread use of contraception has meant that families are smaller than they used to be, and more women are working outside the home. Many women marry in their twenties, have their average two children and go back to work in their early thirties. Their lives are significantly less tied to reproductivity and domestic activities, exposing them to more anxiety-provoking options than ever before, and to all the complexities of social "liberation." However they are still living in a society dominated by male values, a society in which female values are not as yet defined or widely recognized. The various women's movements have played an important part in gaining for women many rights long denied to them, but they have also confused important issues of fundamental values, and agree with each other only in their desire to raise the consciousness and status of women.

Where does the menopausal woman, doubly-disadvantaged by age and sex, stand in this contemporary, ever faster-changing society? She is about fifty years old, so that many of her received ideas are from a different world of thirty, forty, fifty years ago. She started her family or began a career thirty years ago, soon after the end of the Second World War, a watershed in social history; she had her menarche nearly forty years ago, probably before that war started; she was a baby absorbing her mother's milk (figuratively or actually, according to the status of breastfeeding at that time) fifty years ago, and in a very different world. But now she is middle-aged in the world of today, perhaps with a daughter who has an approach to life very different from hers at the same age; and moreover she has a long future of twenty-five years or more in front of her. Paula Weideger comments:

> Women who are sharing this experience [menopause] now, grew up in an era when the definition of the female role accepted by the majority of women—willingly or reluctantly—centred on fertility and motherhood.
>
> In the seventies, despite the heightened expectations of women and the opportunities which have, to some extent, increased, the status and roles of menopausal and post-menopausal women are still being overlooked. When menopause *is* discussed, it is in the socially-acceptable context of its physiological problems. A woman's position in society, however, is less openly considered.[33]

However, in the eighties the problems of middle age and aging *are* being accorded attention by sociologists and psychologists, even if not specifically in relation to women. It is true that the focus of psychologists and others, when upon women at all, is mainly upon the physiological disorders of menopausal women, but their emotional problems have not been completely ignored. Sociologist Pauline Bart, for instance, who studied the phenomenon of depression in premenopausal women, writes:

> Women are more likely now to reach the "empty nest" or postparent stage.... The departure of children is more difficult for women whose primary role is maternal.... Few clear norms govern the relationship between a woman and her adult children. Consequently when the children leave the woman's situation is normless or anomic.... Women whose children leave must also change their expectations, but... there are no guidelines, no "*rites de passage*" for the menopause.[34]

Bart sees menopausal depression as caused by extreme or sudden hormonal decline combined with the identity problems of middle age, some of which are described above. In the American society she was studying there seemed to be a link between the worst depression and the previous intensity of involvement with the maternal role:

> Women who have overprotective or overinvolved relationships with their children are more likely to suffer depression in their postparental period.... Housewives have a higher rate of depression than working-women.... Middle-class housewives have a higher rate of depression than working-class housewives.... The patterns of black female role behavior rarely result in depression in middle age. Often the "grannie" or "aunty" lives with the family and cares for the children while the children's mother works; thus the older woman suffers no maternal role loss. Second, since black women traditionally work, they are less likely to develop the extreme identification, the vicarious living through their children that is characteristic of Jewish mothers.[35]

In the English and Irish groups of women that I have personally observed, there were both similarities to, and differences from, each other and from the American women; but whatever her cultural background, each menopausal woman clearly stands at a crossroads, both in terms of her own change of life and in relation to the accelerating changes in contemporary society.

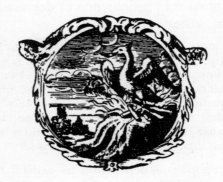

3

Dream-Work in Analysis

Symbolism in Dreams

One of the basic premises of depth psychology in general, and Jungian analysis in particular, is that the unconscious contains a vast amount of information potentially available to consciousness. As Jung remarks:

> Since it is highly probable that we are still a long way from the summit of absolute consciousness, presumably everyone is capable of wider consciousness, and we may assume accordingly that the unconscious processes are constantly supplying us with contents which, if consciously recognized, would extend the range of consciousness. Looked at in this way, the unconscious appears as a field of experience of unlimited extent.[36]

As one kind of unconscious process, dreaming provides the most illuminating evidence we have of our own true states of mind and being—that is, if we can decipher and understand the messages dreams send from the deep recesses of our unconscious minds.

These messages are sent in "code," in symbolic language. It is the same language that the ancients used in framing their myths and religious beliefs. It may originally have been the language of all thought, at a time when there was less separation between the unconscious and consciousness. However that may be, it certainly persists in dreams, and now that we are such consciously rational creatures who "know" so much about the external world in scientific ways, we look at the strange imagery of our dreams and find it incomprehensible.

The first thing people say when they are telling a dream is: "I had such a strange dream last night," or "I just had an amazing dream." Often they find it hard to describe because it appears not to obey the laws of time and space and nature, and can seem to be completely crazy. People who can tell dreams, unworried about the craziness, are often artists of one sort or another. And artists are people who can use symbolism in a way which is organized to express their inner purpose. The insane use symbolic imagery too, but in an uncontrolled and confused way so that they become its victims.

What are these symbols and symbolic events which according to sleep physiologists we dream every night, and which we sometimes remember and find strange? They certainly come out of our minds and, however we disown them, they are our own mental contents perceived by us in sleep.

Jung describes a symbol quite simply as "the best possible expression for a complex fact not yet clearly apprehended by consciousness."[37] Thus a symbol is an image that contains not one but many layers of meaning, "too complex," writes Jungian analyst Rosemary Gordon, "to be conveyed by mere intellectual formulation."[38] The intuitive mind can perceive both the one and the many simultaneously, so that one word or object that presents itself to the senses can burst upon the mind in a shower of meaning, sensation and emotion that has a multiple and moving effect on it:

> The content of a symbol cannot be translated into any other form. On the other hand a symbol can be interpreted in various ways, and this variability of the interpretation, this apparent inexhaustibility of the meaning of the symbol can only be interpreted, it cannot be solved; it is the expression of a dynamic process of thought: it sets ideas in motion and keeps them in motion.[39]

Rachel's first big dream (pages 34-36) certainly "set ideas in motion" for her and for me. The attempted interpretation of its "inexhaustible meaning" and that of subsequent dream imagery, as well as being an important part of her therapy, also formed the thematic link in my study of the menopause.

> The symbol links the strange with the familiar and so forms a bridge between what are really separate objects or experiences. It thus relates the conscious to the unconscious, the here and now to the general and abstract, soma to psyche, physical fact to meaning, the fragment to the whole, and reason to passion.[40]

Jung has said that in interpreting a dream symbol we can

approach it on two levels, the personal and the collective. Sometimes a symbol can be understood only through the personal associations of the dreamer; sometimes meaning can be derived from a universal usage. There are symbols which contain both personal and collective references. Although the concept of the "collective unconscious" is associated with Jung, Freud also, toward the end of his life, expounded a similar theory:

> Dreams may bring to light material which could not originate either from the dreamer's adult life or from his forgotten childhood. We are obliged to regard it as part of the archaic heritage which a child brings with him into the world before any experience of his own as a result of the experiences of his ancestors. We find elements corresponding to this phylogenetic material in the earliest human legends and in surviving customs. Thus dreams offer us a source of pre-history which is not to be despised.[41]

The house in Rachel's dream is an example of a symbol with both personal and collective meanings. It was her own home; the personal associations she brought to it were of the babies she had had in it and the family that had grown up in it and had now left. So on a personal level the house stood as a symbol of her reproductive and family life that was now over. Nobody but she, the dreamer, could know the symbolic significance of the image of that particular house.

Yet she also said: "It was me, my insides, not just my womb," thus indicating that to her the house also represented her body. Now, houses appear in folklore, works of art and dream interpretation all over the world as symbols of the body. They have, that is, a generally acknowledged, collective meaning, and anyone knowing this could have guessed at the significance of Rachel's dream without waiting for her personal associations.

Big and Little Dreams

Jung makes a distinction between "big" and "little" dreams, in terms of their relative importance.[42] Big dreams are the

vivid ones we remember for a long time, dreams that impress
and intrigue us and seem to be pointing a way, to demand
interpretation. They may be sad, happy, frightening or beautiful, but they will not be ignored. Indeed, we should not even
try to ignore them, for they contain information that can be
useful in our everyday waking life.

The dreams of Rachel's that will be presented here were of
such a nature. The first occurred after about a year and a half
of her analysis and we returned to it often. As Rosemary
Gordon points out:

> Analyst and analysand . . . return again and again to the same
> dream, the same fantasy—but with a new insight and with
> some new understanding. For where a symbol operates there is
> always meaning-behind-meaning-behind-meaning.[43]

There are times when dream interpretations are dramatic
and eye-opening. But often they are tentative at first, and the
dream imagery only slowly yields its full significance through
a process of repetition and adjustment. Although there is often
a "click," an immediate apprehension of the fittingness of an
interpretation, clearly there is never any proof of rightness in
a formal scientific sense. The only proof is, as with pudding,
in the eating, and what seems meaningless and indigestible in
the beginning may turn out, as in Rachel's case, to be particularly nourishing.

As for the analyst's part in the interpretation of dreams, this
may vary from person to person, and is a constant subject for
debate among analysts. Personally I feel that the analyst's
intervention should be minimal, and very carefully timed. The
dreamer must be given every chance to describe the dream in
as much detail as possible and to make all possible personal
associations before any interpretation. The analyst can then
contribute ideas based either on knowledge of the dreamer or
on a broad familiarity with symbolic imagery and archetypal
patterns. The effectiveness of the analyst's interpretations is in
any case dependent upon the nature of the relationship between analysand and analyst, and in turn affects it.

PART II

DREAMS AND THE MENOPAUSE

4

Analytic Work with Rachel

Dream One

Rachel had been in therapy for a year and three months before she had her first big dream. When she first came to me she felt that one hour of therapy a week would be enough to "set her on a new path," but two months later she changed to two sessions a week, which she kept up till the end.

She had been surprised to find herself less in control of her own problems than she had imagined; she went through the normal resistance to the material emerging from her unconscious, and was often impatient and angry with me and with the whole process of analysis. In the beginning she brought very few dreams to the sessions, but found that the interpretation of those that she did bring, combined with interpretations of the transference material (i.e., the deeply buried emotional reactions originally projected onto parents and siblings, in later life transferred to other persons and now, in analysis, transferred onto the analyst), gave her significant insights and a hope of progress. About a month before her first big dream she felt herself to be less "in pieces"; she also had a sense of the interior of her body as being a part of her unconscious and involved in the process of growing consciousness.

Rachel's dream had many parts. For clarity and ease of reference here I have numbered the scenes, as she called them. Rachel gave them their titles.

Scene 1: The Burnt House

I am walking round the house in the country, our family home where we all lived when my children were younger. It's burnt out, destroyed by fire, a blackened empty shell. Parts of it look like dead petrified trees, some of it twisted like flames solidified. I am alone...utterly desolate. It's me, my insides, my womb...but not just that...my past life, my children...the whole way of life ended forever...but round at the back of the house there is new grass growing, and that gives me hope.

Scene 2: The Dutch Cap

I am seeing the front part of the blackened and burnt-out farmhouse that was once our home. The front wall has been destroyed, so I see a row of rooms on ground level, open to view like one of those doll's houses where the whole front wall swings back. Each room presents itself like a silent and static tableau, the first of which has the appearance of an oil painting, perhaps of the Dutch seventeenth century. It is a bedroom and on the large double bed lies a woman, not old, not young; she has her head turned away from view, and she has a linen cap on her head. She gives an appearance of fullness, smoothness and maturity. She could be alive and asleep, but I know that she is dead, that she died in the fire, and a feeling of inexpressible sadness and pity comes over me. The overall color of this tableau is a sort of brownish green.

Scene 3: The Dead Babies

The next tableau is in a high barn next to the bedroom. It is not like a painting, but has the tactile quality of real things. The barn is scorched, dry and full of dust and ashes. From the roof hang four twisted dusty ropes, and clinging to them, one on each, are four wisps of what look like fragments of mummified bodies and hair. I know they are children, caught trying to escape the fire. I'm horrified by the gruesomeness and can hardly bear to look.

Scene 4: The Hall of Lost Souls

Next, I am in a vast, dark hall. There are other people with me, being shown around. It may not be my house now but it is still the burnt-out house. On one enormous wall is a great oil painting, perhaps of the Italian Renaissance; it appears to be of a religious subject, not at all clear, but I have an impression of darkness and an imploring figure raising his arms to heaven, where light pours down through a space in the storm clouds and the fierce, white-bearded face of God glares down. There are other shadowy figures in the picture, men and angels, almost lost in the gloom. Then the wall behind this painting swings a little way toward the people, revealing a narrow gap, beyond which is utter darkness. I say to the people, "That's how the fire started. The draft blew through that gap and fanned the flames. It is all the fault of the wicked bosses, who don't care about us."

Scene 5: The Womb-Tomb

Later I am in a tiny, dusty, privy-like room made of greyish planks of wood. There is only just room for me to stand upright in it. It's not really like a privy except for the size—it's more like a coffin, there's no way out, no windows, no doors. I'm desperate, in a panic, I've got to get out. I bash at the wall in front of me; it splinters and breaks quite easily, like an eggshell, and I burst through it into the sunlight at the back of the house.

Scene 6: The Wood Sculpture

It is bright but very neglected, with grass and bushes growing wild everywhere. Then I see in front of me what looks like one rectangular wall standing upright on its own. It appears to be made, not of planks of wood, but of actual branches of trees woven and writhing together. They are of brilliant colors, the orange and red of autumn leaves and greens of grass and trees. Again it is almost like a work of art, a wood sculpture. It is horrific, live trees caught and petrified, flames themselves turned to wood in the act of burning, time stopped forever.

Scene 7: Animus Figures

I am being led away from the house by an eager, smiling clergyman, dressed in a long black belted cassock and a flat, wide-brimmed black hat. He takes my arm and insists I come and see the "foundations." I am irritated and don't want to go with him. It is now very dark. Coming toward us, and going in the direction of the burnt farmhouse from which we've come, are two young priests in black suits. They have black scarves round their faces like masks, with only their eyes showing. I find them enigmatic and slightly ridiculous. Are they priests or gangsters? We pass by each other without any contact, and then the clergyman and I walk into a large field. Over to the right, on a low hill some distance away, I see among trees a large shadowy church or maybe a ruined college building. We are now walking rather gingerly on the red brick wall of the "foundations." This unfinished base of a building is almost entirely submerged in water, with only an inch or two above the surface. As I look down into the water it looks very brightly lit, as if there is a source of light beneath it. I say to the clergyman, "Must you hold my arm and walk beside me? There isn't room for us both, and we'll fall in." But he's smiling and quite impervious. I feel nothing but contempt and am impatient with him, with the "foundations" and with the whole project.

Rachel's reaction to the initial dream-scene, "The Burnt House," was a shock that was almost physical. The impact of the burnt and blackened house and the extreme dereliction of something that had been complete and full of life shook her to the core. Her insight into its meaning was immediate.

The panoramic view of the whole ruin she saw as an image of her hidden physical state at the change of life. She felt the house was her body, essentially her womb; like a "burnt-out case," its contents were dry and dusty, no life-bringing moisture anywhere. She associated the idea of something burnt to burnt offerings and sacrifice; intense heat made her think of hot flushes, and, remembering that Americans called them hot "flashes," wondered if a lightening flash had struck her house and turned it into a cinder.

After Rachel had absorbed the general message conveyed by the burnt house, she turned to the first tableau, the "Dutch oil painting" of the dead woman in bed (Scene 2). She was struck by the fact that though the woman was dead, her body and her bed were the only things apparently not damaged by the fire. In associating to the various images, she came to something like this: the bed was a marriage and childbirth bed, and there was the woman apparently asleep in her place of sex and reproduction, and she was intact. And yet she was dead. She did not show the ravages of fire, she was not blackened or dried up or charred. On the contrary, she was smooth and ripe and brownish green, the color of leaves and grass.

Something did not fit with the rest of the picture, and then Rachel began to laugh. "It's like a Dutch painting," she said, "and she's wearing an old-fashioned linen cap. It's got to be a 'Dutch cap'!" (Dutch cap is the colloquial term in England for a female contraceptive.) She then explained her conflict when she had ceased to menstruate for a year, and was thinking of having her IUD removed. First of all, was it safe? She had not accepted the fact that she was no longer fertile, and, though one part of her was pleased at the thought of the sexual and day-to-day freedom, another part was reluctant to believe that after all these years she could no longer bear a child if she wanted. She thought that the Dutch tableau was telling her that her womb was dead, and she no longer needed to wear her "cap" (IUD).

At the same time, she took comfort from the idea that the rest of her was intact and still alive, still with something of the bloom of ripeness and maturity, not yet withered and shriveled. This was also implicit in the green coloration of the scene, though it was a brownish green, which Rachel associated with a time of drought and autumn leaves.

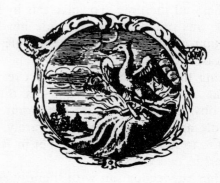

5

The Fear of Knowing

After Rachel had understood and talked through the first two scenes of her dream, some of the "inexpressible sadness and pity" (self-pity) lifted from her, and she thought she was ready to tackle the next part, the gruesome tableau of the barn with the ropes and the withered corpses (Scene 3). In fact, it was a long time before she could bring herself to face up to it. Her mind resisted its message and she became preoccupied with other things—for instance, her eyesight.

In common with most people who have normal sight, Rachel's eyes had started to deteriorate around the age of forty-five, proceeding in the usual fashion so that she needed glasses for reading and any close work. At this particular point in her analysis, she was sure her eyesight was getting much worse and by now was worse than her husband's, although his had started to deteriorate before hers. She was also preoccupied with the problem of making up her eyes, since she could not wear glasses to do this. Another thing that worried her was the awkwardness of spectacles when shopping and in restaurants, etc., when she needed them ready for reading but did not want them all the time. To solve this by hanging them round her neck was practical, but it made her look old. Her husband's solution of bifocals was unacceptable, because they too made her look old.

It is interesting that the deterioration in eyesight generally does happen at around the same time as the menopause. Although it is obvious that both are symptoms of the body's decline in middle age, failing eyesight is rarely, if ever, mentioned in relation to the change of life. Yet in Rachel's case it played a big part in two ways.

First of all, her preoccupation with literally seeing and not seeing came up at a crucial moment in her dream-analysis, when she had just "seen" something that was sad but bearable (the bedroom tableau, Scene 2), and was about to look at something that, at the time, was still unbearable so that she did not want to "see" it (Scene 3, in the barn).

Second was the connection between failing eyesight and narcissism. It seemed more important than ever to Rachel to be able to make up her eyes at this stage of her life, yet her need to wear glasses made this more difficult. At the same time it was important not to look old, not to appear a "fumbling old fuddy-duddy." Also, there was an element of competition with her husband. It seemed he was getting old more slowly than she was and, moreover, the trappings of age were less unattractive for a man. He could have lines around his eyes and wear any kind of glasses, he could look thoroughly middle-aged, and still have an image of distinction and desirability sometimes greater than in youth.

Rachel once said ruefully that Nature did try to be kind: as you got older and more wrinkled, your eyes got dimmer so that when you looked in a mirror you could not see the wrinkles so clearly and could still retain an illusion of youthfulness. Similarly, your peers also appeared younger to you, and you to them. However, most of the time Rachel was unable to delude herself by means of this "gift" of nature. And it was only when things seemed too fearful to be seen, that she did not put on her glasses and have a good look.

The fear of seeing, the denial of knowledge, is in fact an important aspect of any difficulty or crisis to be faced. In *Toward a Psychology of Being*, Abraham Maslow writes:

> From our point of view, Freud's greatest discovery is that *the* great cause of much psychological illness is the fear of knowledge of oneself—of one's emotions, impulses, memories, capacities, potentialities, of one's destiny. We have discovered that fear of knowledge of oneself is very often parallel with fear of the outside world. That is, inner problems and outer problems tend to be deeply similar and to be related to each other.... We tend to be afraid of any knowledge that could cause us to despise ourselves or to make us feel inferior, weak, worthless, evil, shameful. We protect ourselves and our ideal image of ourselves by repression and similar defences, which are essen-

tially techniques by which we avoid becoming conscious of unpleasant or dangerous truths.... (To be completely honest with oneself is the very best effort a human being can make— S. Freud.)

But there is another kind of truth we tend to evade. Not only do we hang on to our psychopathology, but also we tend to evade personal growth, because this too, can bring another kind of fear, of awe, of feelings of weakness and inadequacy. And so we find another kind of resistance, a denying of our best side, of our talents, of our highest potentialities, of our creativeness.[44]

This fear of knowing oneself is particularly applicable to women facing the menopause. Maslow's statement that we tend to be afraid of "any knowledge that could cause us to despise ourselves or to make us feel inferior, weak, worthless, evil, shameful," gives a clue to one reason for this.

The image of the menopausal woman which still today disturbs the unconscious, if not the conscious mind, is of someone who has lost her worth with her fertility, is powerless to attract, is inferior to men and to the young of both sexes, and because of all this is likely to be evil-tempered and unbalanced. What woman would not wish to avoid any thought of approaching this shameful stereotype?

In Maslow's words, "not only do we hang on to our psychopathology, but also we tend to evade personal growth." The concept of development and personal growth is certainly an elusive one for the menopausal woman, when the attitudes of society and her own fears suggest that she has nothing to grow into but the unattractive image described above, an accelerated degeneration of her body, and a slow decline toward death. However, frequently her inner feelings about herself suggest there could be something else, some higher potentiality and, while fear may keep her ignorant of what it might be, there remains the need to know.

I had one other menopausal patient in my practice in Dublin. I call her Marie. She came to me in desperation, racked by a paranoid jealousy toward her husband which had burst out at menopause, and which she had repressed in the past.

Her need was simply to be held, metaphorically, while she poured out her tears of mourning for her lost youth, love and fertility. She never got beyond this stage. Moments of insight were very brief; she resisted knowledge and continually craved support and sympathy as if she could never have enough. During all the time she was with me (nearly two years), she brought only one dream, and it was a clear expression of her terror of knowing. She dreamed that she was walking along a street in Dublin at twilight. It was a poor street that reminded her of her childhood. She passed one doorway, and the door was half-open. She heard loud, violent noises from inside, yet could see nothing, as all was pitch dark. She felt very frightened and ran away down the street.

I tried to work on this dream with her, encouraging her to fantasize about what was behind the door, but she was quite unable to do so. She appeared to be willing, and even to like the idea as if it were a game. But somehow nothing ever happened. No ideas came, she looked to me for help, then her mind went blank or she was distracted by other thoughts. What was behind that door seemed too terrifying for her to face.

The conflict between the need to know and the fear of knowing was also evident in most of the other women I encountered. They were at first reluctant to talk about the menopause, as if talking (except in the most superficial clichés), might bring into being something which could otherwise be denied. Later there emerged a desire to share, to give and take knowledge, and the initial denials could be seen as shields against fear and shame.

6

Narcissistic Mortification

Rachel's preoccupation with her failing eyesight, to some extent related to the fear of knowing, was also associated with narcissism: her fear of losing her youthful, physical attractions, and her need to take even greater pains with her appearance. Psychoanalyst Helene Deutsch writes:

> There is no doubt that the mastering of the psychologic reactions to the organic decline is one of the most difficult tasks of a woman's life. . . . The climacterium is under the sign of a narcissistic mortification that is difficult to overcome. In this phase woman loses all she received during puberty. With the onset of the genital retrogressive processes, the beauty-creating activity of the inner glandular secretions declines, and the secondary sex characteristics are affected by the gradual loss of femininity. . . . We can compare this period to prepuberty. . . . All the forces of the ego are mobilized to achieve a better adjustment to reality, the old values crumble and a drive to experience something new, exciting makes itself felt.[45]

I find this phrase "narcissistic mortification" entirely appropriate to this phase of Rachel's life and to the lives of many other women in the menopause. In view of the increased attention given to the psychology of narcissism in the past few years, by Freudians and Jungians alike, I want to be clear about the way I understand Helene Deutsch's use of the word "narcissistic," and how I am applying it in this context.

The mature Rachel was not normally a narcissistically disturbed person. She related well to others, and had arrived at an adequate, well-balanced view of herself. She had had some early narcissistic problems in growing out of a merger relationship with her mother, whose eye had gleamed a little too brightly and too long at her daughter, but once through the uncertainties of adolescence the more critical eyes of the outside world had modified her self-image.

I believe, however, with Helene Deutsch, that at the menopause there occurs another deep disturbance of the self. It emerges first in terms of appearance, the reflection in the mirror. The literal or apparent image of the self begins to tarnish. Think of the wicked queen stepmother in the fairytale of Snow-White: "Mirror, mirror, on the wall, who in this land is the fairest of all?" She was a narcissistic personality with a vengeance. Her mirror, like Narcissus' pool, had always given her the superlative reply that she wanted, until the fatal day when it answered, "Snow-White is the fairest." At that her narcissistic rage knew no bounds. She smashed the mirror and stormed out to organize the elimination of the dreaded rival who had ousted her and captured the crown of beauty, which is power over men and also the source of auto-erotic gratification between a woman and her reflection.

At the menopause, the marred physical image is a sign of a deeper mortification, a profound blow to the feminine self-image. Now that the woman is no longer fertile, no longer fruitful, what is she? She is not young any more, she is not old; her mothering days are over and she may never again be desirable to men. Her very sense of identity, her feminine self, is threatened.

Rachel and many other menopausal women that I talked to felt this disturbance of the self in a concrete day-to-day way. One woman said, "Sometimes I feel I am twelve years old, sometimes seventy. . . . I feel uncertain how to behave, how to dress, how to relate to people, especially men. How do I seem to them? I just don't know. . . . I never felt like this before."

For some women the awareness of unlived life is almost unbearable. Rachel's very real "narcissistic" pain at this time was at least not compounded by the feeling that the time of her nubility had been wasted. She was able, too, to take comfort from the dream-image of the woman on the marriage-childbirth bed who, in spite of signifying the death of the womb, had "an appearance of fullness, smoothness and maturity."

Nevertheless she found the bodily signs of aging hard to take. She was, against all reason, resentful of her husband whose similar physical decline appeared to have little effect on his sex-appeal. This "unfair" disparity between men and women pained her, particularly as she felt at this stage there was no solution to it. Jealousy was nothing new to her; when she was younger and tied to the children she had at times been resentful of Phil's freedom and opportunities for sexual adventure—but then there had always been a sense of her own sexual power and the possibility of retaliation, whereas now she felt that power to be in decline.

Rachel's transference to me underwent some changes at this time. Her thinking function was highly developed, and for the first year of analysis it had been hard for her to relinquish control of herself during the sessions, to let go of her rational side. The effect of this was to give her an attitude of intellectual superiority. Her mother had been timid and immature, and her father remote, and for a long while she felt unable to trust herself or me with the full burden of her anxieties and fears. This transference of her fragile parents onto me continued until the pressures from her unconscious forced her to test my strength and reality-facing capacity. After that her persona started to weaken, and her self-sufficiency to give way. She began to see me as a woman near her age and to use me as an ally and a support.

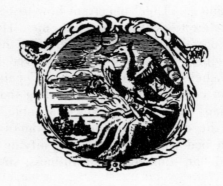

7

Sex and the Menopause

Sexual manners and mores are subject to so much change that it is necessary here to look into Rachel's premenopausal history, and the assumptions of the society in which she was raised and in which her sexual expectations were fostered.

Rachel grew up in England, at a time when a degree of sexual freedom for women was accepted among the small but influential minority of the middle-class intelligentsia, who were her friends and associates. What were the implications of this freedom?

First, it was assumed that women were entitled to sexual gratification and fulfillment. Sex and reproduction were separate functions, and a woman both needed, and was entitled to, fulfilling sex in marriage, and possibly outside of it. This implied the use of contraceptives. It also implied an acceptance of sexual intercourse before marriage and before any permanent relationship was necessarily being considered. There was still a great deal of ignorance among individuals of both the physiological and psychological aspects of sexuality. There was also still a double standard for men and women, although the gap was closing. Promiscuity was frowned upon for women, as was adultery. It was less so for men. A man would still be expected to take the initiative sexually, although a girl would, of course, use all her allurements to bring a man she wanted to this point. Before marriage a girl would expect the man to "take precautions"; after marriage, if they wished to plan their family (which was usual), it was just as likely for the wife to use a contraceptive. (Birth control pills were not in general use until much later.)

Among these emancipated young women of the nineteen-forties, even if reproduction was to be kept out of it, love was considered an important factor in sex, and though a girl might well sleep with several men before marriage, she would very likely convince herself she was in love with each of them at the time.

The Second World War was a factor which gave added incentive to impulsive youthful unions and early marriages, and accelerated the changes in sexual mores which were already in evidence before.

These new sexual mores altered the status of sex in marriage. No longer a marital duty of the wife, sexual intercourse was now expected to be the ultimate expression of mutual passion, and to go on being the major source of mutual pleasure and satisfaction forever. When, in the natural course of events, passion died down and familiarity, domestic routine and other realities of everyday life turned ardent lovers into lukewarm partners or even enemies, the sense of disillusion and disappointment was considerable.

This situation could lead to a serious decline in the whole state of the marriage, at which point there were various courses of action open to the woman. She either ignored her sexual frustration, carried on miserably and hoped it would right itself, or she looked elsewhere for sexual consolation, which was very difficult for a woman with young children, and was incalculable in its effects. Or she would decide she had married the wrong man and would try for a divorce, which sometimes resulted in the same thing being repeated again in another marriage. Or she and her husband could decide to face their problems and disappointments together, and try to work on them. This course of action was a long-term one, and had a chance of succeeding only if there was basic mutual respect.

Rachel and her husband found themselves with sexual problems of this nature in the earlier years of their married and family life. They had married young and each had had one or two affairs before marriage. Rachel described her affairs as "useful experience." In each case she had been physically attracted and had considered herself wildly in love, being temporarily completely obsessed by the man in question. Responding to her own inclinations and curiosity and to the sexual mores I have described, it would have seemed "unnatural," "incomplete" and "unhealthily frustrating" to do anything but go to bed with someone you wanted so much. Although Rachel discovered that she was far from frigid, the sexual experiences were usually disappointing and increasingly so. She put this down to her own sexual immaturity and to the ignorance of her male partners, who were young and comparatively inexperienced. However, Rachel learned from these love affairs a little about men, and a little more about her own sexuality and the way the physical and the emotional were mixed up. She gained a small amount of insight into the mysteries of physical attraction and its apparent evanescence, and also into the balancing of the needs of her body with the needs of her ego.

By the time she met her husband, then, Rachel was somewhat wiser for her experiences, and although their mutual attraction was instinctive and irrational, it was not entirely based on physical attraction. This did not prevent sex from being the focus of their problems in the early part of their marriage, particularly after the birth of their first son. This event classically precipitates all kinds of emotional traumas of an oedipal nature. Rachel was caught between the conflicting demands of motherhood and being a wife, and her husband, jealous of the attention given to his son and withdrawn from himself, felt neglected and insecure and made too many physical demands on her at a time when she was absorbed in the baby. Neither understood what was behind their sexual problems, and for a while Rachel felt that she had made a terrible mistake and that she could never want her husband sexually again. All this was compounded with the usual financial and domestic anxieties that accompany the starting of a family.

Her husband, feeling rejected and needing an outlet for his insulted sexuality and the reassurance that he was loved, had one or two affairs. When Rachel found out about them, she was furiously jealous, especially as she herself would have liked to do the same. There were bad scenes and battles until they realized they were at a crossroads, faced with the choice between increasing alienation moving toward a final split, or working together to try to find out what had gone wrong. With the sad alternative of a prematurely destroyed family confronting them, they both unhesitatingly decided on the second course.

It is hard to realize today, when psycho-sexual and marital problems are so openly discussed and such frequent matter for debate in education and the media, dealt with in explicit detail, both lightly and earnestly, that things were very different in the forties and fifties of this century. In spite of the freeing of sexual mores, the complications arising from living them out had not yet made themselves felt in the public domain; the doctor, the analyst, clergyman and lawyer were available in their varied functions, but rarely resorted to when things went wrong; public sex education as prevention, and self-help psychological groups as therapy, were still in the future.

It is not surprising, then, that Rachel and Phil, who were young when they started their family, were baffled by the problems which confronted them. They had never heard anything about the desired birth of a baby possibly affecting their sexual feelings about each other. Such talk was not in the air. They had both read a little Freud and certainly were intellectually affected by the revolutionary ideas of Freud and his followers, from which no one could remain immune; but they were not able to apply these concepts to their own lives. The oedipus complex was clearly a reality, newly revealed, but it had as yet nothing to do with Rachel, Phil and their baby son. So they decided to go to a psychoanalyst with their problems. As they could only afford for one to go it was agreed that it should be Rachel; she went for two sessions a week. After about four months of this they moved to another area and the analysis had to be discontinued. But as Rachel and her male analyst had built up a good relationship in that time, the analysis, suddenly curtailed though it was, helped to set Rachel on a new path.

She had gained some insight into the nature of her true

feelings about her son and her husband, and one effect of this was to remove blame from both Phil and herself for what had happened. She saw their problems in the larger context of marriage and birth, in a different dimension from the former battlefield of insecure, childish egos, and this removed some of the personal anger and fear. This had a distinct effect on her sexual feelings toward her husband, in some way separating the actual physical excitement and gratification of lovemaking from her emotional resentment and revulsion at his seemingly greedy demands. Because she now recognized the anxiety in his greed and felt less threatened by it and less guilty, she was able to enjoy her body's responses to his, even if she still resented and disliked his mode of approach.

At first Rachel disapproved of this change in herself, as it seemed to go against all the romantic ideas of passionate and total surrender, and to show her as cooly manipulating her own lust at the expense of love. But after a while she abandoned this impractical and utopian self-reproach, since she could see how her new ways were gradually unwinding the vicious spiral of their former sex lives. As she was able physically to respond to him, so his insecurity diminished and he became less sexually overbearing, at which, in turn, her resistance grew even less. There remained for years a memory of the early crisis. It was imprinted on their bodies, and lingered on as an element of "fight" in their sexual encounters, which was perhaps no bad thing since it united rather than divided them.

In middle age, when Rachel looked back over the sexual aspects of her marriage, she felt that the resolving of this serious early crisis was the beginning of a long learning process which would probably end only with death. She believed that the sexual relationship between her and Phil continued as an integral and necessary aspect of their long marriage partnership only because of the art and skills which they had to put into it if they wished for its survival. This implied each of them acquiring some knowledge of their own physical needs and fantasies, those of their partner, the emotional atmosphere in which these fantasies could be acted out and the skill to give mutual pleasure and satisfaction in performance.

It surprised Rachel that all three of these requirements were never actually achieved but were always in the process of development, each interacting with the others. "It's rather like learning an intricate game of skill," she said. When I suggested that this was far from the ideal of marital intercourse as the physical expression of love between a man and a woman, Rachel agreed. But she believed that her idea of it worked and was much more practical. "It is a game in which both partners can become very skilled and well attuned to each other, and it's perhaps best played in an atmosphere of love and ease, although you may only find that out if you change partners for a while." Here Rachel was referring to their various infidelities in the marriage and in particular to a very serious affair which Phil had when they were in their late thirties. After they had come through this painful crisis, their sexual "game" was different again, and, surprisingly, more satisfying than before. Rachel firmly believed that this was because, ever since the lessons of her early marriage, she had been learning not to let the pains and passions of her heart overflow into her sex life, but to preserve that as an outlet for fantasy, a "game of charades."

It seemed from the foregoing that she was able progressively to exert a large measure of control over her own sex life and to find her individual solutions to the problems which confronted her. This situation was due partly to her stable background, which helped to endow her with a balanced temperament and sense of values; and partly to the fact that she grew up in a moderately permissive section of society, which did not intrude or interfere too much with her natural development. She was fortunate in her time and place. A little earlier or somewhere else and her conditioning would have been repressive and inhibiting; a little later and she would have been subject to the consumerist, competitive pressure of modern technological society. As it was, she was able to find, among the other benefits of her background, a great measure of sexual fulfillment as part of a generally fulfilling family life. What were the effects of this at the menopause?

Paradoxically, it was because she had lived, and was living, a satisfying sexual life that Rachel was eventually able to accept the sexual changes and declines she experienced at the menopause. She did not have to grasp after eternal youth, she did not have to pretend to herself that there was "no change." Although not without difficulty, she was able to face the inevitable, including a differently-oriented future. This did not mean that she renounced sex; far from it, but both she and Phil accepted that they wanted sex less frequently than before, and that it was no longer a central preoccupation of their lives. Through this acceptance, they gave practical expression to the idea that "ripeness is all," and that life must be lived in a manner appropriate to the stage of development it had reached.

In Rachel's dream, the tableau of the woman on the bed (Scene 2) provided an image of this idea. The woman was dead on her bed of *childbirth* (Rachel's association); that is, the childbearing part of her was dead—she was no longer fruitful, yet her outward appearance was alive, full and mature as she lay seemingly merely asleep on what was also the *conjugal* bed. Rachel only became articulate and forthcoming about her sexual history when she had worked through to the significance of this part of the dream.

In the 1980s, most menopausal women are living with sexual mores different from those of their youth. The changes have radically affected all of Western affluent society, and although there have been pockets of resistance to change (including Catholic Ireland), the media, and particularly television, have ensured that no part of the world remains unaffected by the so-called sexual revolution. The woman of fifty has to accustom herself to her children's views on sex which are usually different from her own. This is more true today than ever before. Even in Ireland many daughters are using the pill and living with their boyfriends before marriage. In many parts of America and Europe there is a more direct challenge to the middle-aged woman, resulting from the increased pace of technological and consumerist developments in society, from which sex is not immune.

In 1970, Masters and Johnson wrote that "it is widely believed that a postmenopausal woman loses her ability to respond sexually . . . this is nothing more than a cultural fallacy."[46]

The preconceptions were that only young and nubile women had sexual desires and that sex was unthinkable for women after menopause. When the sexuality of a woman ceased to serve both the purposes of reproduction and her husband's legitimate marital pleasure, then any postmenopausal desire on her part was seen as both undignified and unnatural.

Masters and Johnson, and others, gave sanction, then, to the idea that it was perfectly natural and "hygienic" for an older woman to "respond sexually." In other words, her sexual capacity did not end at menopause. This was all very well, but the dissemination of this good news came at a time when it could have some counterproductive effects.

In the American society of Masters and Johnson, and in many European societies of the sixties, everything pertaining to youth and material achievement was worshiped; and sex too was subject to the general gold rush of consumerism. Furthermore, the various women's movements exhorted women to grab their share of the goodies, plus the long-accumulated interest owed to them by an unfair patriarchal society. The older woman was pressured to join her younger sister in the demand for sexual rights, including multiplicity of partners and orgasms, and would have felt inadequate if she had held back. Although the pressures of society encouraged this kind of rat-race mentality, Masters and Johnson had to admit that it was not quite as simple for the postmenopausal woman as they had suggested. They followed the pronouncement quoted above with:

> Administration of adequate amounts of oestrogen reconstitute the pelvic tissues to a state akin to that of the pre-menopausal

years. Given a reasonably healthy male as an interesting and interested partner there is no reason why effective sexual function can't continue for women into the seventy and eighty-year-old group.[47]

There is no doubt that combined hormone replacement can be of great help in restoring the secretions which aid a woman's sexual responsivity, and hormone replacement carefully prescribed can relieve several menopausal symptoms, including those that impede sexual response. But what of the rest of the prescription? Certainly "an interesting and interested partner" might be most therapeutic, but the attempts to prescribe him merely begs the question and rattles the lid of the Pandora's box.

The problem at menopause is not that the woman no longer feels sexual desire, but that her ability to arouse sexual desire in others is waning. It is her feminine power that is at stake, not her sexual capacity. "There are women who know they are capable of enjoying sex, and who are ready to enjoy the intimacy," writes Paula Weideger, "only to find that their mates of years' standing need to find a younger woman."[48]

In fact, the pain and anger brought on by a woman's awareness of the decline of her feminine power in middle age can even increase her apparent sexual desire, sometimes to the point of frenzied promiscuity. It is not necessarily sexual hunger which drives her to this but a desperate need to try to prove to herself that she still has power over men. Weideger points out "the actual facts of life":

> In our culture a woman is sexually desirable only as long as her sexuality can also inspire fear. Once she no longer menstruates she is assumed to have lost her sexuality, but man has lost a great deal of his sexual interest in her—a distinction which is not commonly understood. Men consider menstruating women sexy and menopausal women sexless. Like other male myths about female sexuality, this will go unchallenged as long as women remain ignorant about the actual facts of life. For example, an older woman who finds that her mate is no longer taking sexual initiative may see this decline as proof that she has, indeed, lost her sexuality. But, in fact, this may mean that he is less able to act on his sexual interest than he was when *he* was younger![49]

If one could imagine a less complicated context than that of today, in which the pendulum had swung away from the sexless menopausal image, but not to the other extreme of unchanged, ageless, sexiness, the older woman might in such an ambience be able to age more gracefully and appropriately. She might find, as Rachel did, that if her sex life had once been good, it still could be so, but that her sexual needs were less than before, and her interest in sex was giving way to other preoccupations. She is often afraid to admit this, for fear of not keeping up with her male partner. But he is equally, if not more, pressured to maintain a rampant potency into old age. Although he may still have an advantage in the sexual rat race—in that he can more easily find younger "interested and interesting" partners to stimulate him—he too, if he listens to his aging body's needs, might find they are less urgent than before, and be relieved to slow down in step with his long-time female partner. Clara Thompson's remarks about women also apply to men:

> Many women have a kind of rebirth after menopause. Their general health is better. Freed from concern about possible pregnancy, their sex lives often become more spontaneous and satisfying. Although there is no longer the fiery passion of youth, sex becomes expressive of a tried and trusted companionship and intimacy often more satisfactory in its total meaning than earlier experiences.[50]

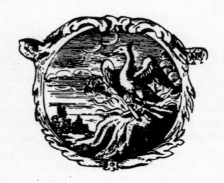

8

Death of the Womb

It was some weeks after Rachel had first recounted her dream that she was able to work on the third scene (the second tableau).

She had faced up to the implications of the burnt house itself, and the first tableau of the sleeping-dead woman on the marriage-childbirth bed, but the spectacle of the room next door had frightened her into temporarily abandoning the dream-work in favor of other matters, such as her eyesight, her narcissistic preoccupations and the sexual competition with her husband. Inevitably, but in her own time, she returned to the dream.

Scene 3: The Dead Babies

> The next tableau is in a high barn next to the bedroom. It is not like a painting, but has the tactile quality of real things. The barn is scorched, dry and full of dust and ashes. From the roof hang four twisted dusty ropes, and clinging to them, one on each, are four wisps of what look like fragments of mummified bodies and hair. I know they are children, caught trying to escape the fire. I'm horrified by the gruesomeness and can hardly bear to look.

Whatever the reason, some of the dread of this gruesome scene had gone and she was ready to associate to the imagery and to amplify her associations.

The four wisps on the ropes, she felt, represented her four pregnancies: three live children and one miscarriage. She "knew" this, first, by the terrible pain of maternal deprivation she felt both during the dream and in contemplating these wisps afterward; second, by a simple verbal association to the "mummified" look of the corpses: mummified = mothered. When she first described them as looking mummified her eyes filled with tears and the connection with Mummy, which the children always called her, and which she called her own

55

mother, became clear to her. The number four at first puzzled her, until she remembered her miscarriage; then she realized that these wisps represented not just her live children but all the fruit of her womb, and that they showed clearly that this fruit was now shrivelled, juiceless, lifeless. They clung to the twisted fiber of the rope like small bundles of scorched and blackened hay in the dusty ash-strewn barn.

"Why in a barn?" Rachel asked herself, and answered the question with her own amplifications: The barn is a granary, receptacle of the ripe grain, the late summer fruit of the fields —a fitting symbol for mature organs of generation, which had not actually germinated and ripened their own seed for many years, but which still remained a storehouse of fruitfulness. But now in the dream this erstwhile storehouse, the barn, was empty of all but its ashes, its dust and its pitiful relics of life. It was no longer the symbol of fading autumnal richness, but of winter barrenness, of death. It was a symbol of the "death of the womb," the end of fertility.

As Rachel became more aware of the message the dream conveyed from the unconscious recesses of her mind and body, she underwent several changes of emotion. First there was the shock to her mind; she felt as though she had woken up from a deep sleep to find that part of her was dead. Then there was an almost physical revulsion, as if the inside of her womb were actually filled with dust and ashes and dry fibers and shrivelled, mummified eggs. Then she felt again the grief of maternal deprivation and was disturbed by it.

"For a moment a terrible pang goes through me, as if I had really lost all my children," she said. "Like the awful things you read about of parents coming home and finding that all their little children have been burnt to death in a fire."

Before the dream, Rachel had not been aware of regretting her lost fertility. She had three healthy grown children whom she loved, and for years she had used contraceptives since neither she nor her husband had wanted more children. She now had a grandchild she could cherish and enjoy, without the ties of responsibility, and was living a life well balanced between interesting work and domestic partnership, and with more freedom than ever before.

"So why should I feel all this pain and regret? It was better before I did all this delving into my unconscious."

When these moments of resentment and resistance passed, she remembered that she had come to me in the first place because everything in her garden was not quite as lovely as she now described it. There was a sense of emptiness, a lack of direction which must have disturbed her enough to make the considerable efforts necessary to go into analysis. She acknowledged this and was able to redefine the feelings she had had then.

"I see now that the feelings I had before starting therapy were much stronger than I admitted or perhaps was aware of. I think I felt hopeless, as if everything was over, it was too late, nothing to look forward to. Yes, as if all hope had been withdrawn from my life and I had no power to renew it."

This last phrase haunted me, as I was to hear the same feelings expressed by many menopausal women. Rachel only knew that she had lost hope and felt powerless to renew it, as she became fully aware that the reproductive time of her life was over. Up to that point she had suppressed the full and conscious knowledge of this bodily fact and its emotional effects. She had only allowed herself to be conscious of the positive aspect of her bereavement (for that is what the death of the womb is)—relief from the responsibility of further pregnancies and freedom from discomfort and inconvenience—and she was reasonably well aware of the other losses of human aging that are shared by both sexes. But the full emotional impact of the one incontrovertible loss for women at the menopause, the loss of the power of reproduction, had remained in her unconscious, unrealized but exerting uncomfortable pressures.

What evidence is there for saying that the hopeless feelings many women have at the menopause relate to the ending of fertility, regardless of their conscious attitudes? My evidence comes from many of the women interviewed but mainly from

Rachel, whom I had the opportunity to observe for some length of time, in great depth, and whose unconscious patterns were revealed through the analysis of her dreams and fantasies.

First, as I have just mentioned, it was only when Rachel truly faced the bodily fact of the final end of her reproductivity that she could fully admit her hopeless feelings.

Second, her phrase, "as if all hope has been withdrawn from my life and I had no power to renew it," made me think of the birth process which produces a new being, a new hope. Fertility is the power to repeat this process; when fertility ends there is no more hope of a new being.

Third, there is evidence from what followed after Rachel's insights. She recognized that the grief and the hopelessness were like feelings of bereavement, and that she was experiencing something like the sad and final loss of a loved one. So, for a few sessions, she mourned her "dead children," her dead hopes. She talked about the little creatures in the barn and wept over them; she remembered in detail her births and pregnancies and her miscarriage; she reminisced over her children as infants and toddlers and had nightly dreams of babies. She savored the deep nostalgia that surrounded the whole generative process from beginning to end: from the moment of knowledge of a new life within, to the tangible joy of a baby at the breast. Then she said farewell to it all. It was gone forever. When this mourning was over she reported that she felt purged of what now seemed to be irrational grief, and she felt ready for what might come next.

As I have said, Rachel was not the only one to report these specific feelings of hopelessness, although because of her dream she was the only one who identified them so clearly with the end of fertility, and was thus enabled to work through the process of mourning for the dead part of herself.

We know that there can be other causes for depression around the time of menopause. In *The Denial of Death,* Ernest Becker writes:

I saw that often menopausal women in psychiatric hospitals were there because their lives were no longer useful. In some cases their role as wives had failed because of a late divorce; in others this circumstance combined with the expiration of their role as mothers because their children had grown up and married, and they were now alone with nothing meaningful to do. As they had never learned any social role, trade or skill outside their work in the family, when the family no longer needed them they were literally useless. That their depression coincided with the time of menopause I thought was an excellent illustration that the failure of useful social role could alone be called upon to explain the illness.[51]

Indeed, "the failure of useful social role" does contribute to depression in middle-aged women. The "empty nest" syndrome and the difficulties of changing roles are considered by many sociologists and psychologists in modern societies to be the main reasons for menopausal disturbance. The solution to such problems is supposed to be that women find new roles in middle age, or, since this is difficult and often impossible, that they never become totally immersed in family-raising in the first place, but have outside jobs from the start which are only briefly interrupted by a strictly limited number of children. Most of the Irish women I spoke to had avoided or at least postponed this particular crisis, by the more traditional method of having large families so that the nest was not empty until much later.

However, Rachel had none of these social reasons for depression; and everything pointed to the fact that her emotional disturbance was caused by the bodily reality of the final shut-down of her reproductive system. I believe too that however they may rationalize, all women are deeply affected by this fundamental change, and the more it is repressed and unacknowledged the more likely it is to cause, as well as depression, many of the morbid physical symptoms often associated with menopause.

In this belief I am supported by the findings of Ernest Becker, who later changed his mind about the "failure of social role" being the only explanation for menopausal depression:

"Role theories" of mental illness ... threaten to abandon the Freudian formulations based on *bodily* facts.... [At menopause] the woman is reminded in the most forceful way that she is an animal thing; menopause is a sort of "animal birthday" that specifically marks the physical career of degeneration. It is like nature imposing a definite physical milestone on the person, putting up a wall and saying, "You are not going any further into life now, you are going toward the end, to the absolute determinism of death." ... Men don't have such animal birthdays, such specific markers of a physical kind. ... But the woman is less fortunate; she is put in the position of having all at once to catch up psychologically with the physical facts of life. ... To paraphrase Goethe's aphorism, Death doesn't keep knocking on her door only to be ignored (as men ignore their aging) but kicks it in to show himself full in the face.[52]

It is extraordinary how apt Becker's words are to Rachel's experience. First, her feeling of loss of direction, of hopelessness, which corresponds to his description of the menopause as a "milestone" saying, "You are not going any further into life now, you are going toward ... the absolute determinism of death." And then came her dream, which was of death in so stark a form that Goethe's aphorism of Death kicking in the door "to show himself full in the face" exactly describes its shocking impact. Then came our work on the scene in the barn, which, we concluded, specifically symbolized the end of fertility, or the "death of the womb" as Rachel dramatically called it. Becker writes of woman being reminded that she is an "animal thing," with the menopause being an "animal birthday." I would find it more aptly called in this context an animal "funeral," but nevertheless it is clear that he meant to emphasize the specifically bodily event that the menopause is. Reproductivity is the female function that women share with all other female animals, and the ending of it is a significant event to be marked like a birthday ... or a funeral.

Becker also notes "how important it is for man to resign himself to his earthly condition, his creatureliness," and then refers to there being no provision in society for the "mourning of one's creatureliness" at the menopause.[53] Rachel spent some time in mourning her "creatureliness" and, as mourning is supposed to do, it helped her to let go of the past and get on with the next stage of living.

9

Anger and Jealousy

Before long Rachel was ready to work on the next part of her dream. Here again is her description of it:

Scene 4: The Hall of Lost Souls

Next, I am in a vast, dark hall. There are other people with me, being shown around. It may not be my house now but it is still the burnt-out house. On one enormous wall is a great oil painting, perhaps of the Italian Renaissance; it appears to be of a religious subject, not at all clear, but I have an impression of darkness and an imploring figure raising his arms to heaven, where light pours down through a space in the storm clouds and the fierce, white-bearded face of God glares down. There are other shadowy figures in the picture, men and angels, almost lost in the gloom. Then the wall behind this painting swings a little way toward the people, revealing a narrow gap, beyond which is utter darkness. I say to the people, "That's how the fire started. The draft blew through that gap and fanned the flames. It is all the fault of the wicked bosses, who don't care about us."

Rachel found this part of the dream very puzzling and she took a long time to work it out to her own satisfaction. She meditated upon it, using association and amplification, and also the gestalt therapy method of identifying with, and personifying out loud, various people and objects in the dream. (Jung has pointed out that every person and thing in a dream can be seen as an aspect of the dreamer;[54] Fritz Perls developed this idea and put it to use in his gestalt therapy dream sessions.) The result of all her work can be summarized as follows:

Although Rachel is still in the same house, it is not her body any more. The intimacy and privacy of the tableau atmosphere has gone. The dark and lofty hall appears to be a public and imposing place, and Rachel is not alone in it. It hardly seems to belong to her any more, but is "open to the public." She is reminded of historic homes and art galleries.

61

The dream seems to have moved from a personal level to the collective or historic level. Rachel's feelings in this scene are different. There is no grief, only a slight resentment at first, and she feels active; she is not the passive sufferer of the earlier parts of the dream. The Renaissance painting is imposing in its size and scope and confirms the feeling of galleries and public places. She notes that Renaissance means rebirth, but as yet this means little to her except the reawakening of her energy and feeling of activity.

The content of the painting introduces a mixture of impressions: a sense of spirituality, but more specifically a sort of orthodox and established religiosity. The weak and helpless human is imploring a fierce, remote old god. The man seems to be at the mercy of both this god and the elements, which swirl darkly around him. Rachel finds in the picture a hint of smug, conventional martyrdom which is distasteful to her. She dislikes the cringing man and the bullying god equally. When the wall swings open and reveals the gap and the blackness behind, this is dramatic and frightening. Rachel feels fear at first and then an increase of her resentment and a sudden anger, as the idea occurs to her that it is the negligence of the "bosses" that caused the fire to spread and destroy the house.

She is reminded of the idealistic indignation of her youth, when she always sided with the underdog, the poor, the persecuted. Now she feels that indignation against men, against the bullying god, the cringing man, the absentee landlords of the dream and also against her husband and her dead father and her sons and all men. She wants to cry out against them as the cause of the catastrophe of her burnt house.

What were Rachel's conclusions about the meaning of this part of the dream? It certainly gave her a different perspective on her menopausal experience, focusing away from the private preoccupation with her own body to something shared and collective. She realized that her anger, directed against men for their neglect of women, was also directed against that part of herself and of other women which colluded with a patriarchal society. She saw the painting as a pictorial representation of that society; the imploring man was the oppressed human being and the god was the old patriarchal oppressor. In so far as she and other people were in society, so were the conventional mores of that society in them; the fact that her unconscious represented the oppressed human as a male made her realize just how much she herself was a part of that patriarchal society, in which many people, including women, were oppressed, but in which the collective human being was always represented as a man, a unit of *man*kind. So the general message was that patriarchal society, of which she was a part, was criminally neglectful of menopausal women, of whom she was one.

There was another group of images in the dream. First, the dark, shadowy and mysterious atmosphere of the hall itself, which was so lofty that the ceiling was invisible; then, in the painting, the man was imploring not only the god but also the elements—winds, storm clouds, raging water. Lastly, through the black gap in the wall blew the winds which fanned the flames that burnt the house. Rachel felt that "elemental" was the word to describe all these images. The dark and mysterious hall felt very different from the earlier bedroom and the barn. In contrast to their "indoorness" and "everydayness," the hall was invaded by the dark and shadows of the night outside. In the painting the little man was at the mercy of the wild elements. And from the black night outside blew the wind that spread the fire. Rachel immediately thought of the "wind of change," and associated all the powerful elemental imagery with the inevitable natural changes which had swept through the dark interior of her own body and dried up its fertility, as the flames had burnt out the house in the dream.

Her unconscious, then, was presenting her with yet another image of her microcosmic bodily changes and their inevitability, this time set within the macrocosmic pattern of natural changes and upheavals, and also within the established pattern of the culture to which she belonged. The final message came to her like this: "Your fertility is ended. This change in you is as inevitable as are the changes in nature of which you are a part. Your anger is against the cultural attitudes toward this change, a culture to which you belong and in which you participate."

For a while Rachel resisted the idea that she was angry with herself, as well as with male-dominated society. In the dream her outburst against the wicked male bosses seemed to express such righteous anger. Everything could be attributed to them; *they* were to blame for the neglect of the beautiful house, the sufferings of "the people," and finally, in their care-less-ness, for the fire that destroyed everything. But, as she came to work on the dream, she had to acknowledge *as her own* every aspect of it. She could not indulge the anger against men, the oppressors, righteous as it may have been, without also owning that she too was part of them (or they an aspect of her), in that she herself had been guilty of neglig-ence and lack of care. Until it came to her own change of life, she had been as thoughtless and as callous toward the prob-lems of menopausal women as was any other man or woman in her society. She thought particularly of her own mother and older friends, and wished they had been able to be more articulate, and she more sympathetic.

Interpreting dreams in this way encourages the dreamer to confront difficult personal truths; in Jungian terms, to face one's shadow. The shadow is the part of oneself one wants to disown. In Rachel's dream-painting, as well as the man and the god there were "shadowy figures ... men and angels," per-haps to remind Rachel that though she might think of herself as being "on the side of the angels," she had her shadow side as well. However, although it was of benefit to Rachel's per-sonal growth and progress in therapy to take responsibility for her own deficiencies, nevertheless her indignation at society's deep-seated negative attitudes toward the change of life was also quite relevant, and bears looking into.

Ernest Becker writes:

We can ... understand how cultural forces conspire to produce menopausal depression in any society that lies to the person about the stages of life, that has no provision in its world-view for the mourning of one's creatureliness, and that does not provide some kind of larger heroic design into which to resign oneself securely.[55]

And again:

Menopausal depression is peculiarly a phenomenon of those societies in which aging women are deprived of some continuing useful place, some vehicle for heroism that transcends the body and death.[56]

The part of Rachel's dream that I have just described certainly indicated an unconscious need for a "larger heroic design" that might "transcend the body and death." It also indicated her anger and dissatisfaction with the design that was there, in herself and in society. Rachel became aware not only of her sense of powerlessness—in her identification with the little human man in the painting—but also of her anger at the bullying godhead and the "wicked bosses" who seemed to be responsible for her deprivation of power.

The strength of this anger surprised her. It seemed irrational to blame men for the natural things that were happening to her. She had always disliked the militant feminists' hatred and hostility toward men, and had rationalized any resentments she may have felt toward her husband and sons, denying that there was any sexist foundation to them. The more the anger persisted and was directed increasingly toward her husband, the more she suppressed it.

Rachel decided that she had done as much as she could with that scene of the dream and so went on to the next:

Scene 5: The Womb-Tomb

Later I am in a tiny, dusty, privy-like room made of greyish planks of wood. There is only just room for me to stand upright in it. It's not really like a privy except for the size—it's more like a coffin, there's no way out, no windows, no doors. I'm desperate, in a panic, I've got to get out. I bash at the wall in front of me; it splinters and breaks quite easily, like an eggshell, and I burst through it into the sunlight at the back of the house.

In spite of the brevity of this scene, it proved to be tightly packed with symbolic material, and provided Rachel with many associations.

But before she could proceed with these, she discovered that the reliving of the breaking-out of the "womb-tomb" unlocked the anger she had been trying to suppress from the previous part of the dream. For three or four sessions she returned to it (Scene 4) and was able to express and amplify her pain and anger at the seeming injustices of the female aging process. In spite of all her carefully built-up defences of a loving marital relationship, her resentments against men in general, and her husband in particular, poured out.

She returned to his infidelities, and it seemed to her that the older he got, the younger the "other woman" got. It was "unfair" that a middle-aged man, even an old man, could go on being attractive to young women. No matter that it might often be experience, fame or wealth that attracted them, to Rachel it seemed a purely sexual advantage that the older man had over the older woman. Every time she read in the press or heard of a case of an older man marrying or having an affair with a young woman, it was a stab in her heart. Sometimes, and it was happening increasingly, the situation would be reversed—a woman in her forties or fifties with a young man. Rachel was consoled by such examples and cherished them, yet in her heart she did not trust them; they made her afraid for the woman, feeling that she was being exploited and was very vulnerable. At the same time she felt anxious about the young man, identifying him with her sons and feeling that he was in some way being polluted by the association.

Many of their friends were divorced. The long-lasting marriages were few and far between. Some of the divorced men had girlfriends or second wives much younger than themselves. When Rachel and Phil went out with them, Rachel wondered if Phil was envying the friend with his young woman.

Most disturbing of all to Rachel was the marriage break-up of a couple who had both been friends for years. The husband, aged fifty-three, immediately married his twenty-year-old girlfriend, who gave birth to a son within a few months of the marriage. Rachel felt this blow to the "old" wife, who was in her menopause, almost as if it were happening to her. She indulged at this point in masochistic fantasies of Phil leaving her and having a baby by a young nubile woman. The pain of these fantasies brought three things home to her.

First, she realized that part of the sexual insecurity she was experiencing at this time was due specifically to her loss of fertility. She deduced this from the particular hurtfulness of the birth of a baby to the young wife. It showed her also that much of the difference between aging men and women lay in the fact that men can retain their fertility into old age.

The second thing the fantasies revealed to her concerned her own sexuality. I called them masochistic and they were truly so in that the pain of them enhanced her own sexual pleasure. When making love with her husband she imagined him as a lecherous old man and herself as a young girl, sometimes matching him in lechery, sometimes resistant—while the part of herself that was the middle-aged Rachel watched, excited by jealousy.

She felt no guilt about these fantasies, which she sometimes shared with Phil and which enhanced their lovemaking. They had agreed that in a long marriage fantasies, whether private or shared, were helpful in keeping mutual sexual pleasure alive. But she began to question what was happening to her sexual desire, and to wonder if she was keeping it on the boil, so to speak, mainly because of insecurity, fear of losing Phil and sexual competition with him. Their relationship was well based on a tried love, mutual respect and shared love of their children. On the rare occasion when they still discussed sexuality, her husband told her that his high-powered, sexually opportunistic days were over, that he was no longer very interested in sex outside marriage, or as a subject for discussion. She trusted him not to treat her badly, but found it difficult to believe that he would be as immune and disinterested as he claimed, if temptation offered itself.

For that reason, and also in response to all the current propaganda on the subject, she had hardly questioned whether she herself was really as interested in sex as she had been in her younger days. Did she any longer crave love affairs, yearn after younger men? Certainly it still pleased her to receive compliments and admiration from men, but that again was a question of security. But did she still have those days when she felt herself to be moving in a haze of desire and sexual arousal?

Up until a few years ago, into her late forties, she had still experienced those days from time to time, and she had observed that they often occurred toward the end of a menstrual period. Although she was aware that a cyclic rise and fall in her sexuality still persisted, she certainly no longer had that heightened sensation. The upshot was that she resented the strain of sexual competition, even though she herself was partly responsible for it. Added to her anger with Phil was anger with herself for continuing to compete instead of trying to find her appropriate sexual level.

The third message that came to her from the unblocking of her pain and anger concerned her relationship with her daughter. In the fantasy of her husband with a young girl, she was either identifying with the girl or she was herself, Rachel, out in the cold, excluded from their erotic dyad and hating them both. As she talked about these painful feelings, she came to recognize the incestuous nature of her jealousy, and to relate it first to herself as the young daughter of her father, and then to her own daughter and Phil. For the first time she faced her jealousy of her daughter, her envy of her youth and nubility, and the painful contrast between her daughter's increasing feminine power and her own menopausal losses.

This awareness gradually released her from the strain of overprotecting her daughter, which she had done up to this point, from her unacknowledged anger. Their relationship became more relaxed and open, and they were able to offer and receive criticism from each other without Rachel feeling that she was attacking or being attacked.

10

Rebirth

Womb-Tomb and Wood Sculpture

Although Rachel had been aware of her hurt and anger when working on the "blame the bosses" dream-scene, she was only able to release it when she had re-experienced her panic in the prison-like atmosphere of the "womb-tomb." Erik Erikson writes:

> The very existence of the inner productive space exposes women early to a specific sense of loneliness, to a fear of being left empty or deprived of treasures, of remaining unfulfilled and of drying up. . . . Clinical observation suggests that in female experience an inner space is at the centre of despair, even as it is the very centre of potential fulfillment. Emptiness is the female form of perdition—known at times to men as the inner life—but standard experience for all women. To be left, for her, means to be left empty. . . . Such hurt can be re-experienced in each menstruation, it is a crying to heaven in the mourning over a child, and it becomes a permanent scar in the menopause.[57]

It took Rachel some time to work through the effects of releasing her anger. They were felt in her family life and in her work as a marriage counselor. Her sexual insecurities, so inevitable a part of the menopausal flashbacks to childhood or adolescence, were not "cured," but by confronting them and releasing the suppressed emotions, she was able to accept them and integrate them into the daily processes of her life. In her analytic sessions she was freed to go ahead with the next stage of her work on the dream.

"I am imprisoned in this dusty little hole," she said, paraphrasing Scene 5. "Ashes and dust are everywhere, and now I am caught forever in the center of my own deadness. There will never be any escape from this dry dead place. It is a coffin in a deserted empty tomb . . . life has passed through this place and left it . . . I scream silently . . . I panic and fling myself against the wall of my coffin . . . it breaks down with surprising ease . . . and I am outside . . . it's the back of the house. . . . "

Apparently she has broken through her "prison" to an area of new life, represented in the next part of her dream as a neglected wilderness:

Scene 6: The Wood Sculpture

It is bright but very neglected, with grass and bushes growing wild everywhere. Then I see in front of me what looks like one rectangular wall standing upright on its own. It appears to be made, not of planks of wood, but of actual branches of trees woven and writhing together. They are of brilliant colors, the orange and red of autumn leaves and greens of grass and trees. Again it is almost like a work of art, a wood sculpture. It is horrific, live trees caught and petrified, flames themselves turned to wood in the act of burning.

Rachel felt this was the climax of her dream, the turning point. If we can see her work with me on the analysis of her dream as a kind of menopausal rite of passage, then this section of the dream would seem to correspond to the end of the ordeal and the beginning of the rebirth process.

Earlier I referred to rites of passage, which have been observed to fall into three stages: first, isolation or withdrawal from society; then the stage of ordeal, involving physical or symbolic renunciation and confrontation with loss and death; and finally the stage of renewal and rebirth after change.

Rachel's coming into analysis corresponds to the stage of isolation, an incubatory experience bringing her closer to nature (her own), away from her usual society and attended only by an "initiated" person (her analyst). Also, during the whole of the first part of the dream she is alone, except for a brief period with an anonymous crowd.

The stage of ordeal can clearly be seen both in the dream itself and in the working-through of its meaning for her. She had to confront the losses of youth, sexual power and fertility, and running through all this was the theme of death, particularly the death of the womb. The climax of the ordeal came, as Rachel said, when she felt herself to be in the coffin, "in the center of my own deadness," trapped in her own dead womb.

Then, after facing her anger and terror, she broke out of the "womb-tomb" (with surprising ease) and emerged into an area of green and growing things and sunlight at the other side of the house from where her ordeals took place. This symbolic birth is clearly the beginning of the stage of renewal and re-entry, changed, into life.

Rachel was not aware of the correspondence between her dream-work and the rites of passage practiced universally to ease the passing of initiates from one stage of life to another. But she was perfectly aware that the dream and our work on it had guided her through a renunciation of a part of her, a painful ordeal, and was now presenting her with a symbolic birth and renewal. She felt a great sense of relief and turned eagerly toward the new, whatever it might be.

The image of the wood sculpture was a puzzle and an obstacle. At first she was disappointed as it seemed to be simply presenting her with more images of wood and fire. She remembered the feeling in the dream, as her relief at breaking out into the sunlight and growing things was changed to fear at the sight of this (yet again) overpowering man-made object. But this time there was an element of exhilaration in the fear, inspiring her to work very hard and persistently. She associated, she amplified, she personified and she used active imagination.

Active imagination is a technique developed by Jung for the clarification or amplification of imagery called up from the unconscious in dreams, drawings, etc.[58] It needs time and solitude and is difficult to do, as it requires conscious awareness combined with a negation of the will, as does advanced meditation. The starting point can be any particular dream-scene or image. One then fantasies oneself into the scene and allows the fantasy to take over, leading wherever it may, with as little willed direction as possible. It is like a waking dream.

I had already mentioned this technique to Rachel. She

seemed to me to have the right balance of "feet on the
ground" (ego strength) and "head in the air" (creative imagination) to benefit from it. She had not attempted it up to this
point, since the imagery of her dream had not seemed to
require it, but now she felt inspired to try. Here is what she
came up with:

> I fantasied myself into the back garden...I am aware of the
> grass, and then I look up to my right and I see this big bright
> hoarding. I walk over to it and stand in front of it, not too
> close. My heart is beating. The sculpture is very still, all the
> writhings and intertwinings of branches and flames are rigid. It
> is all contained in the straight rectangular shape of the frame.
>
> Then the movement and the writhing starts up again...I
> say "again" because I know it had all moved before, and then
> was stopped...It boils and spangles like the shapes you see
> behind closed eyelids. The bright yellow flames and red and
> yellow leaves seem to gather themselves together into the shape
> of a golden bird, huge, hawk-beaked, with wings spread out.
> Then it turns its head and flaps its wings and soars out of the
> sculpture, flying very slowly over the house.
>
> I follow it, not over the house...I wish I could fly but I
> can't...not *through* the house, I think of those horrors...but
> somehow I find myself round the other side, and there is the
> panorama of my burnt home...I am at some distance from it
> now and it looks rather beautiful...The bird comes down with
> a swishing of wings, and lands between two blackened chim-
> neys on what looks like a huge oval grate of wrought iron
> which is full of wood ash and burnt papers. To my surprise it
> makes a loud clucking, just like a hen laying an egg, and then
> ascends almost vertically, flaps its wings and flies off.
>
> A large golden egg lies on the ashes in the grate. I am
> breathing very deeply. Now I am laughing my head off...But
> as the bird flies slowly toward me and over my head I look
> into its stern golden eye...Its head seems to beckon me...I
> take three deep breaths, spread my arms wide and saw them
> up and down in time with the breathing, and then with great
> labor, like rowing against a tide, I ascend into the air, higher
> and higher...I begin to get a feeling of confidence, of being
> buoyed up...I am flying...and that is it...the end of the
> fantasy.

I congratulated Rachel on what seemed to me to be a

genuine product of active imagination. She herself was surprised by it. To begin with she had great difficulty in reaching the layer of consciousness just below will and control; then the outside world "became muffled" and she "got inside" the fantasy. The bird and the way it guided her through the dream landscape amazed her since it had not appeared in the dream itself.

But the question was, did it help to translate the cryptic message of the dream, and in particular did it illuminate the image of the wood sculpture?

The first hints of meaning came from the beginning of the fantasy, when Rachel was standing in front of the sculpture and looking at it carefully. She saw that it represented living, moving things most vividly, and yet was still and contained in a straight and man-made frame. It was a still life . . . a work of art. In this respect it contrasted with the living, growing grass. Then she realized that all through the dream there had been works of art. First the tableau like a Dutch oil painting (Scene 2), then the Renaissance oil painting in "The Hall of Lost Souls" (Scene 4), and now the wood sculpture. It was only now that she put these together and found some new significance in them. To her they represented a kind of creativeness different from the biological creativity of having babies.

The dream had faced her squarely with the loss of that biological creativity, yet indicated three times that there was another way of being creative. Rachel had worked hard on the highly emotive contents of the huge oil painting in the hall, but only now paid real attention to its other message—that it was a work of art of the *Renaissance,* a period of *rebirth.* The wood sculpture itself was an emphatic reminder of the potential brilliance and lifelikeness of man-made creations.

Having already extracted so much meaning from her hard look at the image of the sculpture, how much more could the golden bird show her? Rachel believed that her active imagination had helped her to understand the dream but had also extended and gone beyond it, for she recognized the bird as a phoenix. What she knew about this mythological bird was that it immolated itself in the flames of a fire and arose again intact from the ashes. It was therefore a symbol of rebirth. Rachel did not name the bird during the fantasy, nor had she previously had any conscious thought of the phoenix or what it symbolized. Now, thinking about it, it seemed quite appropriate that a fabulous (man-invented) bird should come out of the sculpture and lead her back to the ashes of the house. (Interestingly enough, Robert Graves describes the word phoenix as "the masculine form of *Phoenissa* (the red or bloody one), a title given to the moon as goddess of Death-in-Life.")[59]

Rachel had already discovered for herself the symbolism of the house, consumed by the moon-fire of fertility and left with a cold and deserted hearth. Now the phoenix descended upon the ashes of this hearth and, having laid its golden egg, rose up again. To Rachel it clearly represented a rebirth, a new self arising out of the ashes of the old. The nature of this renewal had already been indicated by her interpretation of the wood sculpture; further details seemed to confirm that out of the ashes of biological creativity could be born creativeness of a *mental* nature. One of these details was the iron grate upon which the phoenix landed. It was a man-made object, very beautifully wrought, an artifact. The ashes showed signs of burnt papers, which to Rachel indicated the mental activity of writing in progress.

She knew also that the phoenix is a mythic bird of the sun, and in Egyptian mythology its burning and resurrection represented the setting and rising of the sun. The fire of the sun is different from the fire of the moon, which is a smoldering fire, often represented as latent in trees and wood waiting to be brought to life. The bright fire of the sun represents consciousness, mental illumination, the light of reason.

Rachel felt that the golden egg laid among the ashes was a gift from this sun-bird, a gift of hope of a new sort of creative life ahead of her. The banal hen cluckings and her spontaneous burst of laughter Rachel saw as a timely reminder of everyday life and her own nature.

"It's easy to get ridiculous ideas when you're working like this," she said. "You could imagine that you only have to stop menstruating and immediately become a great writer or artist of some sort, that your imagination has no limits. That clucking, the fussy mother-hen noises coming out of that great bird, really brought me down to earth. And when I saw that golden egg, it made me laugh even more. I thought of Mother Goose and traditional English pantomimes."

Thus she confirmed my belief in her balanced nature, which could resist the temptation to become inflated and lose touch with reality, while the feeling of hope and new life remained very much with her.

The last part of Rachel's active imagination concerned her flying. To her this was most important as it gave her new insights, which work on the dream itself had not revealed.

First of all, the technique she employed to get off the ground in the fantasy seemed so real and so possible that she was almost (but not quite) tempted to try it out. In the fantasy it was hard work, requiring a rhythmic persistence of deep breathing and muscular effort which reminded her of giving birth. This labor removed from the whole episode the usual magical ease of dream-flying, and encouraged her to feel that with work and patience she could really give birth to something new. So that when her feet left the ground, and she began to feel buoyant, her delight in the joyous sensation seemed a realistic and possible one.

"For the first time in years I had a sense of real freedom," she said. "I was leaving behind the sad scenes of the burnt house. My children were no longer a burden to me, Phil and I were separate, grown-up people who liked to be together and my parents were both dead. I had never had so few responsibilities to others since I was a child and flew in my dreams. This time I didn't fly so high or so long as I did then, but it was a wonderful moment, a revelation of freedom. I mustn't forget it."

11

Creativity and Individuation

Individuation is a concept central to the theory and practice of Jungian analysis. Jung himself described it as "a process of differentiation [of unconscious contents], having for its goal the development of the individual personality."[60]

The French analyst Georges Verne saw individuation as "a venture which permits the discovery of what is knowable with the help of the faculties at our disposal," and linked it with the intuitive function:

> So long as we use the faculties already known to us, intuition is that part of ourselves which we project towards unsuspected ends; it reveals the reality of what is still unknown and unknowable through creation and mutation. So the unfolding of a life ... is a venture into the unexpected.[61]

Certainly Rachel was caught up at this time in the "unexpected." Her experience was of being born again, and also of giving birth to something new. In both dream and active imagination, these experiences came through the physical sensations of breaking through the eggshell wall and the labor in becoming airborne: the sensation of flying gave to her the experience of the newly born in a different element. Also involved in the experience were feelings of fear and urgency, relief and joy.

As Rachel focused her mind on these events she also became aware of her own creativeness in relation to them. Remembering them and telling them was the beginning of creativity. The next step was to make the connections between them, to link them with other images that emerged from her unconscious into awareness, and by use of her intuition to perceive the beginnings of an integrated pattern of meaning to her experiences. She realized that she had been using these creative faculties throughout her dream-work, but it was only now that she became aware of a surge of creative energy, of excitement and hope. It was for this, she said, that she had entered analysis: to find some way of moving into this next, inevitable phase of life in which she could confront her losses and depletions and find in herself a new and creative individuality.

The term creativeness is meant here in the sense of the ability to link and to symbolize. Creativity is the activity of creating, and a creative person is one who is, in Judith Hubback's words, "psychologically skilled at discerning connection, links of all kinds, symbols of integration and the primary patterns which have an ordering effect in the inner life."[62] All this was true of Rachel.

In a paper entitled "Concerning Rebirth," Jung details many kinds of psychological transformation. Most relevant in the present context is his description of individuation as a process of "natural" transformation:

> In addition to the technical processes of transformation there are also natural transformations. All ideas of rebirth are founded on this fact. Nature herself demands a death and a rebirth. . . . There are natural transformation processes which simply happen to us, whether we like it or not and whether we know it or not. These processes develop considerable psychic effects which would be sufficient in themselves to make any thoughtful person ask himself what really happened to him. . . .
> Natural transformation processes announce themselves mainly in dreams.[63]

The menopause is surely an excellent example of a natural transformation process. In Rachel's case it announced itself in a dream, which caused her to ask what was really happening to her; her work on the dream put her through the ordeal of death and rebirth which Nature, according to Jung, "demands."

The goal of individuation is self-realization. This means establishing a meaningful connection with the totality of the personality, the Self. This individual wholeness can only be achieved through the healing process of integrating into consciousness those repressed unconscious contents which have been traumatic and have upset the psychic balance. "The characteristic psychic processes set in," writes Jung, "the moment one gives a mind to that part of the personality which has remained behind, forgotten."[64]

Rachel was in the initial stage of individuation, and was ready to "move on," to discover and develop her essential wholeness. Would she need first to face the old unhealed traumas, in order to connect with "that part of the personality which has remained behind, forgotten?"

With trepidation, Rachel approached the final scene of her dream. Psychologically speaking, she was feeling the fragility of both the newly born and the new mother. She sensed the obstacles ahead of her, lying in wait, so to speak. Her new resources of creative energy urged her on, yet she feared disappointment and betrayal. She became observably more dependent on me and more anxious that I might let her down. The summer holidays were approaching, her husband seemed depressed. Could she cope with all this newness and the inevitable sorting out of the old? She felt, she said, as if she had moved into a new house, but was sitting on the packing cases amid a wilderness of her old furniture, dreading the task of creating order out of chaos, a new home out of a jumble of old household goods.

She spent a few sessions expressing her anxiety and indecision, testing out her strength and mine, until a day when her confidence returned and she felt ready to retell the last of the dream and face whatever its implications might be.

Scene 7: Animus Figures

I am being led away from the house by an eager, smiling clergyman, dressed in a long black belted cassock and a flat, wide-brimmed black hat. He takes my arm and insists I come and see the "foundations." I am irritated and don't want to go with him. It is now very dark. Coming toward us, and going in the direction of the burnt farmhouse from which we've come, are two young priests in black suits. They have black scarves round their faces like masks, with only their eyes showing. I find them enigmatic and slightly ridiculous. Are they priests or gangsters? We pass by each other without any contact, and then the clergyman and I walk into a large field. Over to the

right, on a low hill some distance away, I see among trees a
large shadowy church or maybe a ruined college building. We
are now walking rather gingerly on the red brick wall of the
"foundations." This unfinished base of a building is almost
entirely submerged in water, with only an inch or two above
the surface. As I look down into the water it looks very
brightly lit, as if there is a source of light beneath it. I say to
the clergyman, "Must you hold my arm and walk beside me?
There isn't room for us both, and we'll fall in." But he's
smiling and quite impervious. I feel nothing but contempt and
am impatient with him, with the "foundations" and with the
whole project.

In retelling this final dream-scene, Rachel was at first aware
mainly of the *feelings* it aroused in her: her intense and physical irritation with the clergyman, which increased with his
bland insensitivity to her reactions; and her uncompromising
and angry contempt for whatever he was offering with such
assurance. This stubborn mood of opposition and resistance,
this absolute certainty of what she did *not* want, struck her as
being unfamiliar in her waking life. I asked her if it was like
anything she had ever felt before.

It reminded her of her anger in the earliest part of the
dream, which had also been directed at established religion, at
"God the Father." Now it was the father-priest, with his solid
foundations and traditional background. I urged her to stay
with the feelings, with the irritation, the opposition and the
contempt.

It turned out that in fact these were exactly the feelings she
had had for her own father when she was an adolescent. She
had felt contempt for what she saw as his conventionality, his
timidity, his acquiescence to authority. She resented the demands put upon her, by both parents, to bow to the same
uninspiring idols. This scorn and resentment frequently put
her into a state of anger which she dared not fully express,
and which manifested instead as constant impatience and irritation. For a time she was "Mary, Mary, quite con*trary*" (her
mother's chant) and totally opposed to everything that was
suggested to her.

There is nothing unusual in this kind of adolescent rebellion, but Rachel felt that her reaction against the parental background was the more violent because she was in fact more than usually immature and dependent upon her home and family. Her older sister apparently grew up and left home with far less conflict. Rachel, however, after three stormy years of needing yet hating her sheltered existence, left home abruptly at seventeen, and never went back except on rare visits.

Between the time she left home and the time she settled down to rearing her own family, she lived and enjoyed a life that, partly consciously and partly unconsciously, was in most respects opposed to her former existence. She rejected the parental values, mores and manners. Her irritation with her parents faded as she saw them so rarely, but her contempt for them and what they stood for remained a long time and never completely left her. It became modified when she had her own children, and gradually over the years she began to appreciate the positive qualities of her early home life: the stability of the first twelve years, the cosily confidential relationship with her mother, the kindness and apparent calm, and later on, even in her difficult years, the noninterference. Even though her parents gave her no guidance in the outside world —and indeed seemed to her unequipped to do so—at least they did not try to stop her going her own way.

This thought brought her back to the dream, and particularly to the possible significance of the male figures in its final scene.

12

The Archetypal Masculine in Women

Rachel's feelings in Scene 7 of the dream were undoubtedly similar to her adolescent feelings toward her parents, and what she was rejecting could be seen as symbolic of the solid conventions and lifeless traditions of her background. Yet the clergyman, though a father-figure, was a stranger and not like her own father. Was he therefore, she asked, an *animus*-figure?- And if so, why was he leading her back to her adolescence, and what was he trying to tell her about her life now? I suggested that she should try the technique of personification in order to find the answer.

The proven usefulness of the technique of personifying dream-objects and dream-figures seems to me to go a long way toward demonstrating the validity of many of the more complex and controversial images which Jung has described as *archetypes of the unconscious.* Among these images are those of the animus and the anima. It was and is not my general practice to discuss Jungian theory or to use specifically Jungian terms in analytic sessions. However, Rachel had a probing intellect and had done some reading in the psychological literature. She was familiar with the concept of the animus and was now interested in its application to herself.

Anima and animus are the terms Jung used for the contrasexual elements in the human psyche. The anima refers to the feminine side in a man and the animus to the masculine element in a woman. The idea of the difference between masculine and feminine ego-consciousness is based on nature, on the difference between bodily form and function, and has persisted through all cultures. Equally persistent has been the idea that men and women carried within them, both consciously and unconsciously, elements of the opposite sexual principle. These elements have been seen variously as gods, demons, soul, spirit, etc., and given names, such as Yin and

Yang, according to culture or religious belief. Freud called this concept bisexuality; Jung saw it as an archetype of both the personal and collective unconscious, and used the names animus and anima for the masculine and feminine images of the archetype. Although ideas of what is masculine and what is feminine have undergone many changes, and in spite of contemporary feminist protests that any differentiation is discrimination, there are eternal truths based on the facts of nature. June Singer expresses this reality as follows:

> It is evident that what is qualitatively different about The Creative and The Receptive is the Masculinity of the first and the Femininity of the second, and what is equally important is that both of these qualities are present in the intrinsic nature of each human being regardless of sex. These qualities are not necessarily culture-bound or culturally conditioned, as some contemporary sociologists assert, except in so far as the trends of society follow the necessities of Nature. . . . When this Masculine archetype [The Creative] becomes manifest in a woman, as it surely does, it needs to be recognised as the fertilizing "other." This Jung saw when he called this archetype *animus,* meaning the Masculine element in the psyche of the female. . . . Men are born with a penis which simply and naturally is used for penetration, while women need to develop their phallic potential in order to *penetrate the world.*[65]

It is interesting that Rachel had complained in so many words that her father had not helped her to "penetrate the world." The clergyman in the dream, however, seemed to be trying to fulfill just that animus function. After much work of amplification and personification, Rachel came to the following conclusions.

The clergyman is hurrying her away from the burnt family house, and busily getting her interested in something entirely new. This new thing is connected with traditional education and established religion. The clergyman reminds her of a Canon Jones who used to visit the headmistress of her boarding-school and sometimes take prayers. The school was built of red brick and had "solid foundations," both physically and metaphorically. Her college, too, was a similar Edwardian building. Her father was keen on her having this sort of conventional education.

The clergyman, then, she saw as that masculine part of herself that wanted to succeed and gain recognition in the solid world of the academic establishment. He wanted to get her away as quickly as possible from the old feminine-reproductive life that was over, and he paid no heed to the protestations of the feminine part of her. He was an animus-figure from her unconscious, derived partly from her father and partly from the teacher-priest image of her schooldays. His interaction with her in the dream represented a conflict within herself. She could see that the conflict referred to her present stage of life and its problems of adaptation to a new sort of creativeness; but she was disturbed by the apparently immature behavior of the dream protagonists, which made her feel the confusion and insecurity of her adolescence.

She had hoped that her animus would prove to be the perfect spirit-guide into the future, instead of a "narrow-minded, boring, insensitive old fool with conventional ideas." Her anger turned toward her father, whom she blamed for being the representative of masculinity branded on her impressionable young mind, molding the configurations of her animus. What she needed and lacked now were the masculine qualities of thrust, initiative, originality, daring.

She then realized that her husband had these qualities. She had been instinctively attracted to him because of this dynamic quality which contrasted with the cautious stability of her father. As she and Phil inevitably changed with parenthood and the years, she had come to recognize and appreciate the complementary nature of their relationship. While their children were growing up it was fine that he should have the aggression and determination needed for the intense competition of the outside world, leaving her free to develop her feminine side in the home. But now it seemed to her that they had become rather too polarized in their masculinity and femininity. She had relied too much on Phil's dynamism, and because of it she had never developed her own "phallic potential." Against all reason she felt angry with him again, as if *he* were responsible for depriving her of the power she needed to go forward, and for leaving her with an inadequate animus image.

She was brought back by these associations to the overdependency of her adolescence, and the anger and humiliation she had felt because of it. It seemed that the scars of this time had never quite healed and now were making themselves felt again. Men were always building walls around her and protecting her from the world, but the walls made a prison as well as a shelter.

Recent experience had shown her that anger was needed in order to break out (e.g., the womb-tomb in Scene 5 of her dream). Now perhaps anger would arm her for the unknown world outside. Hitherto, her reason and her sense of guilt (both well developed) had curbed the full expression of her anger. Now she let go with streams of abuse against her parents and her husband. Murderous fantasies that had been concealed by overanxious death-fears were exposed; the culmination was a fantasy of the clergyman drowning in the water surrounding the foundations, overbalanced by his own clumsy eagerness.

At the end of this, she felt no sense of forward progress toward independence or self-realization; but neither did she feel any longer her former disappointment with her interior animus-figure. With the release of anger, she became reconciled to him. Instead of expecting too much (the perfect guide), she accepted him as he was—just one of many changing forms of her animus. If he were as yet inadequate to guide her, then for the time being she would have to rely more on her femininity. Her focus had shifted. She did not feel pressured to follow a linear route to individuation, but experienced herself more as looking around and waiting. There were other animus-figures in the dream and, meanwhile, she felt stronger and calmer. The desperation of the newly reborn had left her.

Psychoanalyst Pearl King, writing about the treatment of

older patients, emphasized the importance of accepting destructive impulses, as well as loving ones, toward those people
we consciously love and value. This enables us to see and feel
toward them as whole people (i.e., not split into good and
bad) with their own separate existence, feelings and point of
view, etc., and not as extensions of ourselves.

> If this stage has not been satisfactorily reached in the course of
> life up to adulthood, individuals find it very difficult to accept
> and integrate (without falling ill) the sequence of losses and
> depletions that ageing and death inevitably confront them
> with. It offers the possibility of working through the guilt and
> bitterness of life's failure, and gaining enrichment thereby.[66]

Rachel's confrontation with the clergyman animus-figure in
her dream, and with the anger resulting from it, enabled her
to withdraw many of her animus projections from the real
men in her life. She began to see that she had projected onto
her husband the positive masculine qualities which she herself
needed. He did in fact possess them to a great extent (i.e., he
was a good "hook"), but, like herself, had other sides to him
and problems of his own; he did not exist only in order to
complement her and to prop up her weaknesses. She had
always known this with her head, but now she understood this
aspect of their partnership and began to relate to her husband
in a more realistic and psychologically objective way.

For some years Phil too had been going through a mid-life
crisis. Each of them had tried to show goodwill toward the
other and to be sympathetic to the other's problems, but their
mutual unconscious projections made this difficult. Lately, as
Rachel moved toward more independence, Phil had been
showing signs of strain and depression. The rationalization
they both accepted was that it was the usual "male menopausal" crisis of waning potency, expressed in Phil's case
mainly in terms of career-fatigue and disillusionment, and fear
of the up-and-coming younger men.

With her new sensitivity to Phil as a "whole person" with a
"separate existence," Rachel now realized that while his creativity at work was central, it was intertwined with his uncon-

scious needs of, and demands on, her. She observed (and remembered it had happened before), that with each step of hers toward independence, he was affected in some way. He might become ill, or irritable or depressed, and the effect on her was a feeling of guilt and a temptation to step back. She now saw that he was as ambivalent about her independence as she was. In one way it was a threat to him. Her dependency had kept her bound to him, as it had to her parents; it meant she was always there to minister to him (as his working mother had *not* been). His protection of her was thus also a protection of himself and the family.

But as they all grew older, the strain of maintaining the protective walls increased, and by the time they had reached their present stage, he was torn between a desire to have a strong woman who could keep him (a standing joke between them), and the old infantile fear that such a woman would just get up and leave.

Emma Jung, the wife of C.G. Jung and herself an analyst, wrote about the nature of the animus and the anima:

> The character of these figures is not determined only by the latent sexual characteristics they represent; it is conditioned by the experience each person has had in the course of his or her life with representatives of the other sex, and also by the collective image of woman carried in the psyche of the individual man, and the collective image of man carried by the woman. . . .
>
> Just as there are men of outstanding physical power, men of deeds, men of words, and men of wisdom, so, too, does the animus image differ in accordance with the woman's particular stage of development or her natural gifts. This image may be transferred to a real man who comes by the animus role because of his resemblance to it; alternatively, it may appear as a dream or phantasy figure; but since it represents a living psychic reality, it lends a definite coloration from within the woman herself to all that she does.[67]

Rachel's experience corresponded with all these points. The original animus image, derived from her experience of her father, she had supplemented with a rather more heroic image derived from the collective unconscious; this she had projected onto her husband, who came nearer to filling the heroic role. As Emma Jung writes:

> We try with real cunning to make the man be what we think he ought to represent. Not only do we consciously exert force or pressure; far more frequently we quite unconsciously force our partner, by our behavior, into archetypal or animus reactions. Naturally, the same holds good for the man in his attitude toward the woman. He, too, would like to see in her the image that floats before him, and by this wish, which works like a suggestion, he may bring it about that she does not live her real self but becomes an anima figure. This, and the fact that the anima and animus mutually constellate each other, ... forms one of the worst complications in the relations between men and women.[68]

Rachel spent some sessions sorting out Phil's problems from hers, his anima projections from her animus projections. Then she returned to the dream-scene, where she now saw her animus presented in yet another form, that of the two young men.

The first important factor seemed to be that while she was being hurried away from the house by the elderly clergyman, the two young priests were walking back in the direction from which she had come. But who were they and what did they mean to her? Why was one animus-figure leading her one way while this mysterious pair went the opposite way? They had priesthood in common, which suggested to Rachel "spiritual guidance," as well as the negative personal associations with the clergyman. But the boys were also "gangsters" and seemed rather dangerous; at the same time, they looked slightly ridiculous. Rachel felt as attracted to this enigmatic pair as she had felt repelled by the other, and her inclination was to follow them. Then she had a sudden and vivid personal association.

At her mother's cremation nearly two years before, she had stood in the chapel with her two sons, one on either side of her. At the awful moment when the coffin started to slide inexorably toward the opened doors and into the furnace, Rachel was stricken with grief. Her sons moved closer to her, each taking an arm. She felt great strength and support from them. Earlier on, before the funeral service started, she had noted their strange appearance in very similar dark suits. Normally dressed in jeans and sweaters, they had all found the funereal garb somewhat ludicrous. Her sons were the same height, and, dressed alike, they gave the impression of an almost identical clerical pair.

This association released a flood of emotion and later understanding. The animus was truly functioning as, in June Singer's words, "the fertilizing other."

The two dream-figures were leading her back to the burnt house, symbol of her dead motherhood. They were like her sons who had given her strength when the body of her dead mother was burning, and perhaps like those heavenly twins Castor and Pollux, who represented respectively mortality and immortality. Her sons were not normally seen in a religious setting, dressed like clerics. Usually they looked more like cowboys in their jeans, boots and leather jackets, and were busy fighting for a living in the competitive outside world. It was that aspect of Rachel's son-image which was expressed by the gangsters' black face-scarves.

Her attraction to these figures was based on the remembered feeling of loving strength coming from her children, at a time when she was poised in middle life between the death of the old generation (and her own powers of generation) and the vital growth of the next (her first grandchild was a month old). This young strength supported her and helped her forward, away from the past and into something new.

Yet the dream seemed to indicate that the "something new" derived from the youthful and positive animus was to be found back at the house. This was an enigma to Rachel; she wondered if anything had been forgotten, if there was "unfinished business" connected with her family relationships.

The emotional release which these memories of her mother's funeral had triggered had already brought about one change in her life. She had become close again to her younger son. For some years there had been a hiatus in their relationship. There was no quarrel or even coolness, but they seemed to have very little to say to one another. She had called it noninterference, and "letting him get on with his own life." Ever since he left home and she had had no active mother-function toward him, they had both withdrawn almost to non-communication. Rachel had noticed the same change in the relationship with her older son when he no longer needed her mothering. But it had not been so extreme and had changed again when he got married and started his own family. She had decided that she and her younger son were too alike, in that they were both introverted and inclined to be withdrawn, and so she had accepted the static condition of their relation-ship, telling herself that this was what it meant to let one's children go.

She now discovered that it was possible to get close to him again, to talk and laugh together and to exchange ideas. Their encounters, whether frequent or rare, were warm and dy-namic, as in the old days. Her son's response clearly indicated that he felt no need to defend his privacy by anxious with-drawal; on the contrary, he was released by her initiative, and seemed free to express his feelings or not, as he felt inclined. Rachel now understood that she had simply lacked the "phal-lic power" to penetrate his world. Consciously experiencing her animus had given her the creative power to break the deadlock that had stultified their relationship.

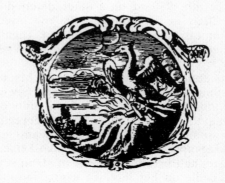

13

Integration of the Feminine

Dream Two

It is evident from the foregoing that Rachel was deeply moved by her first big dream and by the re-experiencing of it in her analytic sessions. She accepted its ultimate unfathomability as a manifestation of the mystery of her increasing self-realization, which was already changing both her inner and outer life in subtle ways. Nevertheless her intuition told her there was yet a further depth to be reached.

After her work on the animus-figures in the last scene of her dream, Rachel and Phil went on holiday and visited their family. Soon after they came back, Rachel had another big dream:

> I am fourteen or fifteen at the beginning of the dream. I go to my sister Betty's bed-sitter [one-room apartment] to look for her. She is a college student about eighteen years old. I very much want to see her, but she's not there. A nondescript, shadowy woman of about forty-five, perhaps a maid, says Betty had a party last night and she is out at the moment. I feel hurt that she didn't ask me to the party and disappointed that she's not there.
>
> Then I'm outside walking on a quiet, deserted quay by the sea. There is Betty in her little car. I'm overjoyed to see her and I get in the car. She seems pleased too. Then she changes and becomes cold and critical. She wants me to get out of the car.
>
> In the next scene I am my present age. My daughter has told me something about having a baby, and how she is totally resentful and unforgiving toward me. I am guilty of everything bad happening to her, and all is over between us. She is departing for somewhere by train and I am below on the platform looking up at her. She is not like herself; she looks like a half-caste (half-breed) black girl of about seventeen. She has a vicious smile on her face, an expression of triumphant hate. I am angry and tell her so. But as the train moves off, I feel only terrible grief and despair.

It was clear to Rachel that this dream was about her personal relationships with all the women in her life, and also about her own femininity, constantly changing. Although her mother did not appear in the dream, "her ghost was haunting every scene," said Rachel.

In the first scene Rachel is a young girl, not yet a woman. Her sister, older by three years, is past puberty and has all the pleasures and privileges of grown-up womanhood: a place of her own, parties, her own society, etc. Moreover, the maid, an older woman, also seems to belong with Betty. The young Rachel is excluded from the sisterhood of women who menstruate, to which both her mother and her older sister belong. The middle-aged maid is the dreaded image of the nondescript, redundant, menopausal woman that Rachel sometimes feels herself to be in relation to *her* student daughter enjoying her own youth in a bed-sitter. This scene reminded Rachel of forgotten feelings of early adolescence, when her mother and sister really did seem to belong to something from which she was excluded. She longed to start menstruating and, until she did at fifteen, felt ashamed of her immaturity.

This early attitude was a very important aspect of Rachel's whole approach to menstruation and to everything else to do with her reproductive function. She welcomed the menarche so wholeheartedly as her entry into womanhood that she never experienced problems with menstrual periods. On the contrary, apart from the occasional inconvenience, she enjoyed her periods, finding that they gave her a special feeling. It was hard to describe: a quiet, inward-turned, melting feeling, rather as if she were sitting alone in front of a fire with a sleeping kitten curled up in her lap. She felt self-sufficient, inclined to reflection, meditation. She was not aware of this at every period, and there were times later, when she had a family, that she felt tense before and tired during menstruation, but she never suffered the pains and miseries during either periods or pregnancies that she heard about from other women. A passage in *The Wise Wound* puts the menstrual cycle in a perspective she could appreciate:

Menstruation is regarded, not only by physiologists and many doctors, but also by some feminists, as a sickness, a blank spot, a non-event that the women must endure and would be better without, an evil time. This simply is not necessarily so. It is the time when the healthy woman may draw on abilities and capacities that are not related to the values of ovulation and childbearing, but that are instead related to that other side of her nature, of independence of thought and action. It is the exact counterpart, but in an opposite sense, of the ovulation. At ovulation she wishes to receive, accept, build, if she desires a child. But from menstruation there is a different set of energies available to her of receiving, accepting, building *the child which is herself.*[69]

The second scene was very brief in action and condensed in meaning. It took a great deal of work and attention to detail.

She happily gets into her sister's car. She has joined the sisterhood of women, and is welcomed into it. The car is a symbol of adulthood and independence, which they now share. It is also the sheltering womb from which they both came. Then everything changes. Her sister is cold, critical and rejecting. Rachel must get out of the car and walk on her own.

This brought back to Rachel the disillusionment and pain of growing up and growing apart. She remembered that she had expected, when she was sixteen and thought of herself as a young woman, that she would share her sister's wonderful world. But Betty believed she was spoilt by their mother, and had always been jealous of Rachel. She didn't want her young sister intruding into her world and perhaps stealing her friends as she had stolen her mother. Rachel became aware of this as she identified with her dream-sister. The tensions and rivalry between them had simmered over the years without either open warfare or real reconciliation. They lived far apart, and saw each other rarely.

Rachel now realized that things had become worse between them a few years ago, when her sister must have been in *her* menopause. Betty had been aggressive and resentful. There was a brief mutual warmth and sympathy at their mother's funeral, although shortly after that event there was an atmosphere of recrimination resulting in Rachel's intensified guilt about her mother.

The setting of this dream-scene on a quay near Dublin provided other associations, all connected with separation. When Rachel came by boat to Ireland some years earlier, she left behind all her family with the exception of Phil and, for a short time, her daughter. She felt no emotion at leaving her sister, married and with a family of her own. But parting from her boys and from her aged and widowed mother was an ambivalent process.

The quay at Dun Laoghaire reminded Rachel of the guilt she felt about leaving her mother, and also of Betty's renewed resentment at being left with the responsibility of their mother's final years, while Rachel "got away."

From this recent memory of her sister's cold criticism, Rachel associated back again to yet an earlier parting when she had left home at the age of seventeen, avid for "independence," which had somehow not arrived automatically with the onset of physical womanhood. Growing up was more of a struggle than she had realized, and people got hurt. First she herself was hurt, and then she hurt her mother. Now she remembered how cruelly she had kicked her way out of the sheltering home which seemed to smother her.

This memory of her own cruelty took her into the next scene of the dream, in which her daughter is unmercifully cruel to her and seems almost to be glorying in her own hatred. She says something vague about having a baby and blames Rachel for everything bad that has happened to her.

Although the intensity of the negative emotions in this scene were distressing and apparently alien to Rachel, her associations came rapidly. She identified with the daughter, remembering her own anger with *her* mother for failing to equip her for life, particularly sexual life. She had been eager to become a woman and to experience sexual love, and her mother, taking for granted her virginity until marriage, had left her in ignorance of all practical details of sexual intercourse and of avoiding conception. She had had to learn everything by experience, and though she had been lucky and avoided disaster she felt terribly vulnerable, as if she had set out on the most hazardous of journeys prematurely and ill-equipped. In the same way, her mother had seemed unable to prepare Rachel for the birth of her first baby; she herself had apparently been unconscious throughout her deliveries. Again Rachel learnt through her own first experience and prepared herself far better for her subsequent childbirths, which were "natural" and therefore less painful and more conscious experiences.

Through these memories, Rachel came to realize that her contempt for her mother had grown steadily from prepuberty on. Before that time they were very close, often like sisters. At that stage, her mother's immaturity and dependence on her husband had the effect only of creating a cosy and undemanding nursery atmosphere. But as Rachel grew up she needed something more, something her mother was incapable of giving. On the contrary, she clung to her younger child, and thus started in Rachel the inevitable cycle of fear of dependency leading to rejection behavior, leading to guilt and remorse.

She now knew that she had asked from her mother what it was impossible for her to give. "I wanted her as I grew up to be quite a different sort of woman from the mother I loved as a child. I wanted a worldly mother, a sophisticated woman, wise in the ways of men and of the world. It wasn't a very conscious wish, but for a time I projected it onto my older sister, and it certainly affected my choice of friends from the age of thirteen on."

As more understanding came, Rachel realized that she had failed to appreciate fully the positive aspects of her mother's femininity. As far as her personal limits allowed, her mother had enjoyed being a woman and, particularly, being a mother, and never conveyed any of the negative attitudes toward her female biology and psychology that were, and still are, so widespread among women. She was almost invariably gentle with her daughters, overestimating their talents and strengths as they grew up, so that gradually she seemed herself to become the younger sister or daughter. This confusion of identities is echoed throughout the dream.

What of Rachel's own daughter in the dream? She appears

to be about seventeen, the age at which Rachel left home. Rachel associated her daughter's cruelty in this scene of parting to her own cruel rejection of *her* mother. But there is more to it than that.

It is *her* daughter who is going away and leaving her bereft, and *she,* Rachel, is now suffering the grief of a rejected mother. Although Rachel had suffered some pangs as her daughter grew up and left home, and though she had recently been made aware of her jealousy of her daughter's youth and nubility, there had been nothing in their actual relationship to explain the intensity of her emotions in the dream.

Rachel associated the train moving slowly out of the station with her mother's coffin gliding out of sight at the crematorium. Then she had grieved that the finality of death had deprived her of the forgiveness and complete reconciliation which her sense of guilt demanded. The feeling of despair at the departing daughter in the dream was certainly similar.

But there was something else that eluded her, something between her daughter and herself that she found difficult to approach.

The clue was in the image of the daughter. She was "not quite herself," in fact she looked like a half-caste black girl. Rachel had no personal associations to a half-caste, so she thought that the image must represent half her daughter and half something else. A black girl suggested an alien, or opposite aspect.

It has been observed that for whites, the images of black people in dreams or fantasies normally have a collective significance. If devoid of any personal associations, as in Rachel's case, they usually stand for something primordial, instinctive and mysterious, perhaps a primitive force.

Rachel felt that the cruel, half-black girl was a witch, something out of hell, dancing in triumph on the coffin of her (Rachel's) youth, and that this was an eternal aspect of the daughter for the mother. "My daughter reminds me of my own dead youth; and also of my cruel young self leaving *my* mother in tears."

The strangeness of the dream-daughter conveyed to Rachel

the idea that she was experiencing an aspect of the mother-daughter relationship which went beyond the personal, and was in fact an archetypal feminine experience.

The archaic Greek myth of Demeter and Persephone confirms her intuition. Persephone was the daughter of Demeter—a goddess associated with fruitfulness and mature womanhood—and Zeus. At Zeus's instigation, Earth lured Persephone away from her friends by means of beautiful narcissus flowers. As she stooped to pick them, Earth opened up and Hades carried her off against her will into the underworld. Demeter, stricken with grief, wandered the earth searching for her lost daughter. She heard that Persephone was in the underworld and went to Eleusis, disguised as an old woman, to plead for her return. Meanwhile, in despair, she used her power to prevent any crops from growing on earth until Persephone was found. Zeus finally persuaded Hades to give Persephone back to her mother. Hades, however, by giving Persephone a pomegranate seed to eat, ensured that she would return to him; it was agreed that she would spend a third of the year in the underworld and the rest on earth with her mother. Demeter caused the crops to grow again and commanded that a temple be built at Eleusis, where her rites were celebrated thereafter.

These rites, called the Eleusinian Mysteries, were celebrated in Greece for two thousand years from about the middle of the second millenium B.C. As well as representing the natural cycle of the death and rebirth of vegetation, the Mysteries also illuminated aspects of the feminine experience through the mythic story of mother and daughter. Essentially matriarchal in their nature, the Mysteries died out as patriarchal values became dominant, but the myth remains, and, since Rachel's dream is so resonant with its themes, it is worth extracting what meaning we can from it.

Nancy Carter, exploring the meaning of the myth in connection with Margaret Atwood's novels, writes:

Demeter is seen as the ripe grain, Persephone as the tender shoots; together they are invoked as the "two goddesses." In

The Great Mother, Erich Neumann speaks of the two as "virgin and mother [who] stand to one another as flower and fruit, and essentially belong together in their transformation from one to the other." Furthermore, Neumann names the *heuresis,* the "finding again" of Persephone by Demeter, as the one essential motif in these and all matriarchal mysteries. Not only does the "finding again" signify annulment of the male rape but it also re-establishes the nuclear situation of the matriarchal group; the primordial relation of daughter to mother is renewed and secured in the mystery. Persephone's sojourn in Hades also signifies fascination with sexuality, the male earth aspect; the appearance of the narcissus and the pomegranate, one phallus, the other seed, reflects this idea in the myth.[70]

The mother-daughter problem, both in the myth and in Rachel's dream, involves their necessary separation and mutual transformation. The daughter must leave the mother in order to fulfill her nature, join herself with a man and become herself a mother. The mother would like to keep her daughter with her always, as she would like to keep her own youth perpetually in flower. Hades represents not only the Male who lures away the daughter by playing on her own nature, but also Death, *which threatens* the fruitfulness of the mother.

Just as Rachel had experienced the integration of her masculine side through the animus-figures in her first big dream, so in this dream she experienced profoundly her femininity as both mother and daughter. She was particularly shaken by the confrontation with her daughter as a creature from two worlds, one black, one white, departing from her forever—or so it seemed.

14

Separation and Transformation

Dream Three

As Rachel proceeded with the dream-work and relived the pleasures and pains of her womanhood, she could feel the beginning of a healing process taking place. The point of departure in the dream, the bidding farewell to the daughter, was itself a starting point of a new return. At that point she experienced herself as a woman in "the change of life," parting from her childhood, her girlhood and her motherhood. But as she relived the experiences of her earlier life through the figures of her mother, her sister and her daughter, and mourned their ending, they became a part of her again in a new and more conscious way. "I feel I have grown, or rather filled out. There is more of me. I am a more *considerable* person."

Not only did the dream-work restore to Rachel these aspects of herself, by a process of integration, it also restored to her real-life daughter, sister and dead mother their integrity as persons separate from her. It caused a discernible change in the way she related to them. She saw her daughter with a new insight, and was able to give love to her as a separate person, confident that their natural separation was not rejection. The guilt she had felt toward her own mother, which had increased after her death, virtually disappeared, leaving only intermittent regret that she had not understood more when her mother was alive.

Rachel now saw a new meaning in the mysterious pair of priest-gangsters who in the first dream (Scene 7) led her back to the family house. They incorporated the young male priests of Eleusis serving for a season the mother Demeter, goddess of birth, death and rebirth; and also the immortal Hades, seducer and fructifier of the daughter Persephone. By leading

her toward an integration of her feminine aspects, they enabled her to strengthen and deepen her feeling relationship
toward men (an important animus function).

Like the celebrants of the Eleusinian Mysteries, she began
to feel the psychological benefits of the reliving of her myth-
like dream. It was as if she now had her own substance and
her own space, that is, her individuality, and yet belonged
more than ever to the human race. She remembered the dim,
middle-aged woman, who "might have been a maid," in the
first part of the dream. She saw this figure as "a typical
menopausal image" which she had feared to resemble: shadowy and nondescript, hovering uncertainly around the periphery of other people's lives, with no home or place of her
own. Now she saw another side of this figure which she
associated (rather apologetically) with me, as one whose function was to "hover" there, acting as messenger or link between
conscious and unconscious.

In the analytic sessions Rachel now began to express herself
in an emergent, outgoing way. She noticed for the first time
objects in my office that had been there all the time; she
asked my advice about expanding her work-skills; she talked
increasingly about her life outside. There was a new warmth
and closeness with Phil and at the same time a greater feeling
of autonomy and freedom, as she became less involved with
his changes of mood. She visited her daughter in college and
they had a wonderful time, with none of the tensions she had
expected.

The ambivalent attitudes of impending separation (from
me) began to show themselves in our sessions, until one day
she came with a "final" dream:

> I am my mature self, sitting in an armchair in a spacious room
> of what seems to be a club. There are other chairs around,
> forming a circle. Opposite me is sitting Angela, my oldest and
> best friend. We are talking and at ease with each other. A
> group of men enters; they remain standing and talking among
> themselves. One of them comes toward us, smiling. It is Jamie
> McDonald, an old friend of mine from college, who became an
> actor. I haven't met him since university. He looks as he used

to, about twenty-two years old. We are happy to see each other. It appears I have had a wonderful idea for a project, perhaps a play or performance of some kind. Jamie is delighted with it and the other men move toward us and are friendly and congratulatory. I am surprised, they seem to know more about it than I do. Then I remember that I have not introduced Angela and she may feel left out. But she is not at all offended, calmly smiling and taking part in the general conversation, sharing the atmosphere of pleasure and appreciation.

Rachel and her friend Angela had grown up together from the age of thirteen. There was a close bond between them, in spite of long separations over the years, and the fact that they had very different personalities. Rachel instinctively chose her as a friend for the qualities of independence and worldly wisdom she had wished for in her mother and which she thought she observed in Angela even at that early age. As they grew up their relationship became more equal in terms of sophistication, but Angela retained her independence in that she earned her own living after leaving school and kept herself and her one child without financial help from a man. Her marriage to a rather weak and ineffectual man had broken up after six years, since when she had had many affairs but had never remarried. Her son had grown up and married, and she lived alone.

Rachel therefore regarded Angela as representing in the dream a sort of alter ego: a mature woman like herself, but with opposite qualities; focused on work and not on family; free where she was dependent; insecure where she was protected. Their being together and talking comfortably in the dream suggested to Rachel a reconciliation of opposites within herself, an expression of her psychological integration.

The setting of the armchairs in a club atmosphere meant to Rachel the "club of women" or sisterhood in which she now felt like a fully paid-up member. This was the feeling of "belonging" to something almost impersonal, larger than oneself or family. She and Angela together formed an integrated personality, that is, her former qualities reinforced with Angela's independence and worldly competence. (Of course she recognized that the real-life Angela was, like everyone else, an incomplete person, with the problems of her own deficiencies.)

The figure of Jamie McDonald produced interesting associations. The group of men with whom he came into the room seemed to Rachel to be that aspect of her animus which represented the collective masculine world outside the home and family. But what did Jamie himself mean, presented so vividly by her unconscious after thirty years of no contact?

She remembered that Jamie had acted even at college, and was prominent in university drama productions, always playing lead parts. As she described his activities, she became aware of all the "masculine" associations to the words she was using. He was an "actor, acted, was active," "was prominent," "played the leading man." Furthermore, he had once urged Rachel to take part in a play he was producing. Although interested in drama she had never much wanted to act, but allowed herself to be persuaded by Jamie to go to an audition. She failed to get the part, and afterward Jamie gave her his opinion of why this had happened. He told her that she had spoken her audition piece with feeling and intelligence, but that somehow it was too small and private to come over to the audience. She lacked *projection*. If the decision was solely his, he would have given her the part and taught her how to project herself, how to magnify the small sensitive performance so that it forced itself upon the audience's attention. Rachel, a little dashed by the whole experience, felt sure he would not have been able to produce this transformation, and was relieved to be able to retire into backstage obscurity. However, the incident had lingered in her mind as a piece of potential self-knowledge which she was unable at that time to understand fully or to apply.

Now it seemed the dream was telling her that the transformation had happened. She *was* capable of "projecting" her personality outward. Her "project" was apparently highly acceptable. She had gained the attention and support of the outside world of men for her performance as a woman. This performance of a woman's role was effective because of the integration within her of the many aspects of her femininity, combined with the masculine elements revealed by her dream-work.

There was yet another dimension to the dream. The two women in armchairs reminded Rachel of her analytical sessions, during which she and I sat talking in comfortable chairs facing each other. I was now, in contrast to the former image of the faceless servant, a friend and equal in "the club of women." The change in the nature of our relationship is also reflected in Rachel's anxiety in the dream about neglecting the Angela-me figure, and the reassurance that she (Angela-me) was in fact getting on perfectly well with her own conversation and was not feeling rejected.

This told me that Rachel sensed that she could now get on in the world without me, and had needed to reassure herself that *I* would be all right without *her*. The ending of an analysis is indeed a delicate process which, like other separations, needs time and sensitivity to accomplish without trauma. I was grateful for the signs of Rachel's awareness of both her strength and mine, and of her readiness for our separation in an ambience of mutual caring and respect.

Rachel's analysis came to an end some six weeks later. As is usual in the course of an analytical relationship, I had learned a lot about my patient and something new about myself. In these pages I have focused chiefly on the dream-work and Rachel's progressively deeper insights, but our transference-countertransference exchanges, referred to here only briefly, were also an important factor in her analysis. After she left I became aware of having played at least three roles in the final significant nine months: as constant companion and support; as guide exploring and opening up new paths into life; and also as spectator and follower, often in awe and wonder of a transforming journey that was in fact already beginning for myself.

Conclusion

The experience of accompanying Rachel's individuation process was a revealing one, made even more so by its close, step-by-step correspondence with that natural transformation of body and soul that takes place at the change of life.

What did we learn about the menopause? Certainly my researches in the literature gave new information, and taught me facts about the menopause which every woman should know, but few of us do. Yet these facts (which Rachel called "the facts of death"), together with information on the so-called management of the menopause, *are* available, if sought for, in sensible books and booklets written for the public by women doctors and others.

Why then are so many women of menopausal age ignorant and evasive (as both Rachel and I had been) about the changes ahead of them? Perhaps more of us would be able to confront the realities of aging and move positively into the future, as Rachel did, if the attitudes of society did not make it more difficult.

In early societies where female fertility was worshiped, there is little evidence that there was an important role for the *post*fertile woman; and in later patriarchal societies the fertile woman was seen to have a dangerous sexual power, which concentrated ceremonial attention and ritual controls upon her, again leaving the postmenopausal women in an insignificant and apparently ignored position. The power that the menstrual taboos imparted to nubile women remains in the unconscious even today, and the image of the bereft, menopausal woman is with us still; she is either Rachel's colorless dream-figure, hovering at the periphery, hoping for a useful role, or she is flushed and neurotic, moody as an adolescent but without the freshness or the promise.

Thus women's own fear of the consequences of losing youth and nubility, compounded by society's age-old neglect of the postfertile woman, has deprived the menopause of meaning

103

and the menopausal woman of dignity. Yet, if the fears and taboos were lifted, how could the menopause *not* be recognized as a significant life-passage? If the beginning of reproductive life is recognized as crucial, and if the fruits of reproductive life are celebrated, how can the ending of it not have deep meaning, at least for the women concerned? There is a great need here for the understanding and support of a life-change as crucial as puberty or the first childbirth.

The societal situation today is ambivalent; while on the one hand the statistics of life expectancy have made the post-menopausal woman a force and presence to be reckoned with, due to sheer numbers, and while older women are now therefore important consumers in a consumer society, nevertheless these societies worship youth and productive achievement, regarding the aging and aged as so much unproductive ballast. Even as it becomes more difficult for society to ignore the elderly, it can and does continue to neglect and undervalue the special qualities and the creative potential of later life, and particularly the later life of women. Women's movements have until recently shown no special interest in the older woman. Their solution to women's problems in general has been for them to take every opportunity to live and work as men in a man's world; thus reproductivity and family life lose importance, jobs and careers gain importance, filling a woman's life and eliminating as far as possible specifically feminine biological roles, changes or problems.

The more recent interest in the older woman (in the United States there is a movement called OWL, for Older Women's Lib) appears to have merely extended this "solution": the older woman is still encouraged to feel that the menopause is a non-event, but one which happily enables her to be more than ever like a man, and, with the help of life-long hormone replacement, to beat her overstressed male contemporaries to the top jobs, while remaining younger, healthier and sexier than they. In other words, the "solution" seems to be to stay in the endless sexual rat race.

Rachel's dreams revealed a different pattern. They showed

that the menopause, far from being a non-event, was one of great significance to her as a woman. Through the dream-work the process of her menopausal experience laid itself out like a blueprint, with which it became possible to compare the menopausal processes of other women.

The first common theme to emerge was the "fear of knowing and the need to know," manifested in Rachel and in all other women wherever I talked to them. This ambivalence toward acknowledgment of the reality of the menopause is a manifestation of the fear and shame women feel as a reflection of historic neglect, set against their present need for information and the sharing of ideas and feelings.

The dream-work showed Rachel that "the facts of death" were about loss of youth, loss of feminine sexual attraction and loss of fertility, and that all these losses were hard to bear.

Menopause is connected with aging, and aging implies the approach of death; this is why women do not want to think about it. But menopause is much more specific than that. Men also have problems of aging, but they do not literally lose the power of renewing life, as women do. With the loss of fertility women lose also much of their power of sexual attraction, if not of sexual capacity.

There is an enigmatic significance about the loss of reproductivity that cannot be denied or explained away. First, it is the one loss among those mentioned that belongs, without doubt or argument, to the menopause. Yet why should a modern woman in a modern society be disturbed by it? Why should she not rejoice at her freedom? Rachel asked herself the same questions when her dream presented her with images of her dead womb. She had had all the children she wanted and for years she had been actively preventing more births, yet she felt grief at her involuntary and perpetual barrenness, as if at a personal bereavement. After full acknowledgment of her feelings and a period of mourning, she was all right and could go on, even savoring her freedom from day-to-day parental responsibilities. What she had mourned was her own *fruitfulness;* the very word seems to make the grieving understandable, in spite of all the rational denial. The other women I met, even many of the Irish mothers of big families, expressed relief at the end of fertility but also sadness that something was gone forever.

That phrase, "gone forever," brought home to me again the symbolic significance of the end of fertility. As well as the actual conceptions, pregnancies and births that may have shaped the realities of her life, the woman of fifty has lived for thirty-five years or more with the monthly repetition of the potential to create new life. Whatever her conscious attitude or her unconscious reactions toward this cycle, it inevitably represents the constant power of renewal. At menopause that power ceases, and to the menopausal woman it seems at first that hope has gone forever, it is too late, the future is empty.

As the end of a lifelong rhythm, then, the change of life requires of her that she learn to live from day to day and rediscover her creativeness in a new direction. That is the task and that is the future.

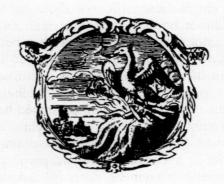

Postscript

Every woman has her questions. What really happens? Will I change, go crazy, dry up, get wrinkles, grow frigid? Will I become like my mother? Will my husband want me? Will any man? What can I do? Should I take hormones? Do they help? Are they safe?

Mostly these questions are unspoken. Each woman's menopause, when she comes to it, is a deadly secret, cannot be told, must be hidden—out of sight, out of mind—got through as well as possible with nobody knowing.

Because of this conspiracy of silence, menopausal women do not talk easily, do not willingly share their experiences and help each other.

In the last few years, there *has* been more information available; more books and more articles written, more menopause clinics, more self-help groups where information can be shared, more medical research into hormone replacement. Information *is* there and that is important. But information is not always reliable. Medical information, for instance, is constantly changing, often going into reverse, invariably controversial within the medical profession itself.

Information is hardly ever unbiased. Bias in information can arise from the prejudices and attitudes of even the most well-meaning informant.

For example, Wendy Cooper's book, *No Change,* is packed with information on the menopause. It is reliable and based on careful research, but her prejudice shows in the title. She sincerely believes, and presents the evidence to support her belief, that hormone replacement is so effective that it can, and should, virtually eliminate "the change." This is her attitude, the philosophy that lies behind the information she gives.

All of us seeking information are equally biased. We are looking for the answers that will satisfy our secret hopes and wishes. The most universal of these is the wish for eternal

107

youth. Menopausal women are particularly vulnerable to this one. Behind all the questions is the faint hope that "the change" could be "no change," that estrogen could be the elixir of life and hormone replacement the fountain of eternal youth. This vain hope is encouraged by the mass communications of our consumer society, which insistently sells success and happiness as the byproducts of youth, beauty and sex-appeal.

Like every other adult in this society, the menopausal woman has to sort out for herself the most balanced advice from the conflicting information presented to her by pundits and experts. She can do this most effectively if she is supported by a positive attitude toward herself during the change of life, an underlying philosophy of life that can make of the menopause a progressive experience, in spite of conflicts and uncertainties. It is not in vain attempts to ignore the changes of age and to pursue the trappings of youth that strength and happiness for the older woman lie. On the contrary, that way leads to bitterness, exhaustion and instability. Even more destructive is a masochistic surrender to the inevitability of woman's "sad lot," a lifelong conviction that female biology has always been the scourge of women, and that the menopause is the final blow; that kind of feminine defeatism leads only to debilitation and decline into premature old age.

On a practical level, Rachel, like many other women, took advantage of available information. When the hot flushes became uncomfortable, she sought medical advice, and on the basis of that advice made her own decision to take the new (at that time) combined natural hormones. They eliminated the symptoms after two months, at which point she stopped them, and subsequently repeated the treatment when the symptoms reappeared. Because she had no illusions that hormones would make her young again, she was thankful for their specific effectiveness, which improved her well-being and facilitated her sexual response.

In spite of such "good management," she still found herself in the emotional state of emptiness, hopelessness and confusion that prompted her to come to me for psychological help.

Once she had acknowledged the need to "open the cellar door" to her unconscious, her dreams revealed to her not only the symbolic representations of her fear, grief and anger, but also those hidden sources of healing and renewal within that could lead her toward a fuller realization of herself, a real change of life. Ursula Leguin describes the process:

> There are things the Old Woman can do, say and think which the Woman cannot do, say or think. The Woman has to give up more than her menstrual periods before she can do, say or think them. She has got to change her life. . . .
> The woman who is willing to make that change must become pregnant with herself at last. She must bear herself, her third self, her old age, with travail and alone. Not many will help her with that birth. Certainly no male obstetrician will time her contractions, inject her with sedatives, stand ready with forceps and neatly stitch up the torn membranes. It's hard even to find an old-fashioned midwife, these days. That pregnancy is long, that labor hard. Only one is harder, and that's the final one, the one which men also must suffer and perform.
> It may well be easier to die if you have already given birth to others or yourself, at least once before. This would be an argument for going through all the discomfort and embarrassment of becoming a Crone. Anyhow it seems a pity to have a built-in rite of passage and to dodge it, evade it and pretend nothing has changed. That is to dodge and evade one's womanhood, to pretend one's like a man. Men, once initiated, never get the second chance. They never change again. That's their loss, not ours. Why borrow proverty?[71]

Each woman's experience of the menopause will be different, but if we can assimilate the shadows of the past and accept the realities of aging, it may be found that the menopause, though a difficult and demanding passage of adulthood, can also be a time of psychological integration and growth, increased strength and specifically *feminine* wisdom.

Vital ingredients of such wisdom are wit and humor, attributes not usually associated at the present time with the postmenopausal woman, but ones which traditionally represent a liberating factor in her life. In many societies the old woman was given a degree of license that was forbidden in her fertile years. She could join in with the men, tell bawdy stories and generally release her libidinal energy from many of the restrictions society imposed on the nubile woman. This increase of freedom was accompanied by greater self-confidence and authority in the society outside the home, and in some cases a sanctioned domination over men. Such a situation does still exist in the American South.

> Many of the women who tell vile tales are gloriously and affirmatively old. They transcend the boundaries—not by their station and employment—but by aging beyond the strictures that censure would lay on the young. The South, like many traditional cultures, offers an increase in license to those who advance in age, and ladies I have known take the full advantage offered them in their tale-telling. They seem to delight in particular in presenting themselves as wicked old ladies.... As the Southern Black comedienne Moms Mabley used to say: "Ain't nothin' no old man can do for me 'cept bring me a message from a young man."[72]

Spinners of tales, teachers of the young, healers, midwives, dressers of corpses, celebrants of rituals, wise and wicked, the older women "are specialists in those critical moments, when the designs of culture are threatened by a breakthrough of nature—birth, illness and death—moments when we are reminded of our animal origins and human limits."[73]

There is much talk these days of racism, sexism and even agism. We so fear negative discrimination that we blur the differences which so richly and meaningfully distinguish one group or individual from another.

Age differences *are* important. Aging brings experiences the young cannot dream of. The young experience life in a way the old do not, but the old can and should remember, and know how they have changed. One of the most vital people I know is a woman of eighty-four who is still fascinated by her life day by day as it unfolds, and still learns from it and likes to share her insights. She can hardly remember her menopause, but she says she always found changes stimulating, she had raised five children, it was time for something new. She recollects that it was then that her "time-sense" grew up: "I stopped looking forward for something wonderful to happen, and learned to live today, this minute." Since then she has had another full lifetime of thirty years.

The menopausal experience of Rachel and the post-menopausal lives of such women are well worth studying; they constitute the best kind of information a woman can find as she faces change and uncertainty. They—and her own dreams—may even provide answers to her unspoken questions.

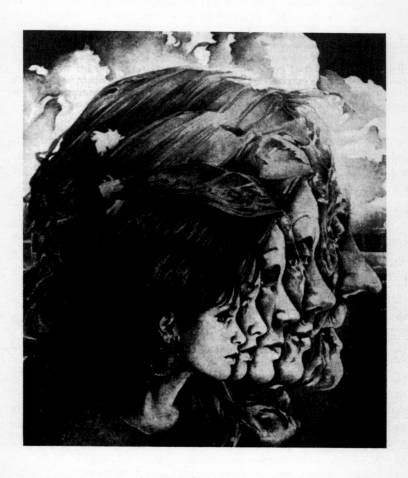

Notes

CW—*The Collected Works of C.G. Jung*

1. C.G. Jung, "General Aspects of Dream Psychology," in *The Structure and Dynamics of the Psyche*, CW 8, par. 488.
2. Joseph Campbell, *The Hero with a Thousand Faces*, pp. 8-9 (italics mine).
3. Abraham Maslow, *Toward a Psychology of Being*, p. 60.
4. Helene Deutsch, *The Psychology of Women*, vol. 2.
5. E.g., Esther Harding, *Women's Mysteries, Ancient and Modern*, and Erich Neumann, *The Great Mother*.
6. Mircea Eliade, *Myths, Dreams and Mysteries;* Joseph Campbell, *The Hero with a Thousand Faces* and *The Masks of God*.
7. James George Frazer, "Taboo and the Perils of the Soul," in *The Golden Bough*.
8. Margaret Mead, *Male and Female*.
9. Wendy Cooper, *No Change*.
10. Paula Weideger, *Menstruation and Menopause: The Physiology and Psychology: The Myth and the Reality*.
11. Rosetta Reitz, *Menopause, A Positive Approach*.
12. Penelope Shuttle and Peter Redgrove, *The Wise Wound: Menstruation and Everywoman*.
13. E.g., Matriarchy Study Group, *Menstrual Taboos;* Susan Lipschitz, ed., *Tearing the Veil;* and Barbara Ehrenreich and Deirdre English, *Witches, Midwives and Nurses*.
14. Shuttle and Redgrove, *The Wise Wound*, p. 27.
15. Bernice Neugarten, "A New Look at the Menopause."
16. John Studd, "Management of the Menopause."
17. Ibid.
18. See Arnold van Gennep, *The Rites of Passage*, a classic account of initiation rituals in primitive societies.
19. Campbell, *Hero with a Thousand Faces*, pp. 10-11.
20. Cooper, *No Change*, p. 59.
21. Robert G. Richardson, *The Menopause: A Neglected Crisis*, quoted in ibid., p. 64.
22. Shuttle and Redgrove, *The Wise Wound*, p. 142.
23. Weideger, *Menstruation and Menopause*, pp. 218, 217.
24. Elaine Morgan, *The Descent of Women*, pp. 257-258.

25. Mead, *Male and Female,* p. 180.
26. Weideger, *Menstruation and Menopause,* p. 216.
27. Pauline Bart, "Depression in Middle-aged Women," in *Women in Sexist Society,* ed. V. Gornick and B.K. Moran.
28. Vieda Skultans, "The Symbolic Significance of Menstruation and the Menopause," pp. 639-651.
29. Shuttle and Redgrove, *The Wise Wound,* p. 228.
30. Ibid.
31. Harding, *Women's Mysteries,* pp. 127ff.
32. Diagram Group, *Woman's Body: An Owner's Manual,* p. 194.
33. Weideger, *Menstruation and Menopause,* p. 209.
34. Bart, "Depression in Middle-aged Women," p. 136.
35. Ibid., pp. 214-215.
36. Jung, *Two Essays on Analytical Psychology,* CW 7, par. 292.
37. Jung, "The Transcendent Function," in *The Structure and Dynamics of the Psyche,* CW 8, par. 148. See also his lengthy discussion in "Definitions," *Psychological Types,* CW 6, pars. 814ff.
38. Rosemary Gordon, *Dying and Creating: A Search for Meaning,* p. 108.
39. Arnold Hauser, *Social History of Art,* quoted in ibid.
40. Ibid., p. 107.
41. Sigmund Freud, *Outline of Psychoanalysis,* p. 28.
42. Jung, "On the Nature of Dreams," in *The Structure and Dynamics of the Psyche,* CW 8, pars. 554ff.
43. Gordon, *Dying and Creating,* p. 110.
44. Maslow, *Toward a Psychology of Being,* pp. 60-61.
45. Deutsch, *The Psychology of Women,* vol. 2, pp. 456-457.
46. Masters and Johnson, *Human Sexual Inadequacy.*
47. Ibid.
48. Weideger, *Menstruation and Menopause,* p. 220.
49. Ibid., p. 219.
50. Clara Thompson, *On Women,* p. 171.
51. Ernest Becker, *The Denial of Death,* p. 214.
52. Ibid., p. 215.
53. Ibid., p. 216.
54. Jung, "General Aspects of Dream Psychology," in *The Structure and Dynamics of the Psyche,* CW 8, par. 509.
55. Becker, *The Denial of Death,* p. 216.

56. Ibid.

57. Erik Erikson, "Womanhood and the Inner Space."

58. See Jung, "A Study in the Process of Individuation," in *The Archetypes and the Collective Unconscious,* CW 9i, pars. 622-623, and "The Transcendent Function," in *The Structure and Dynamics of the Psyche,* CW 8. Also Barbara Hannah, *Encounters with the Soul: Active Imagination as Developed by C.G. Jung.*

59. Robert Graves, *The Greek Myths,* vol. 1.

60. Jung, "Definitions," in *Psychological Types,* CW 6, par. 757.

61. Georges Verne, "Individuation and the Emergence of the Unexpected," p. 35.

62. Judith Hubback, "Reflections on the Psychology of Women."

63. Jung, "Concerning Rebirth," in *The Archetypes and the Collective Unconscious,* CW 9i, pars. 234-235.

64. Jung, "A Study in the Process of Individuation," in ibid., par. 619.

65. June Singer, *Androgyny,* p. 199 (italics mine).

66. Pearl King, "Notes on the Psychoanalysis of Older Patients."

67. Emma Jung, *Animus and Anima,* pp. 1-3.

68. Ibid., p. 11.

69. Shuttle and Redgrove, *The Wise Wound,* pp. 30-31 (italics mine).

70. Nancy C. Carter, "Demeter and Persephone in Margaret Atwood's Novels: Mother-Daughter Transformations."

71. Ursula Leguin, "The Space Crone," quoted in Marta Weigle, *Spiders and Spinsters,* p. 195.

72. Rayna Green, "Magnolias Grow in Dirt: The Bawdy Lore of Southern Women," quoted in ibid., p. 194.

73. Barbara Myerhoff, "The Older Woman as Androgyne," quoted in ibid., p. 192.

Glossary of Jungian Terms

Anima (Latin, "soul"). The unconscious, feminine side of a man's personality. She is personified in dreams by images of women ranging from prostitute and seductress to spiritual guide (Wisdom). She is the eros principle, hence a man's anima development is reflected in how he relates to women. Identification with the anima can appear as moodiness, effeminacy, and oversensitivity. Jung calls the anima *the archetype of life itself.*

Animus (Latin, "spirit"). The unconscious, masculine side of a woman's personality. He personifies the logos principle. Identification with the animus can cause a woman to become rigid, opinionated, and argumentative. More positively, he is the inner man who acts as a bridge between the woman's ego and her own creative resources in the unconscious.

Archetypes. Irrepresentable in themselves, but their effects appear in consciousness as the archetypal images and ideas. These are universal patterns or motifs which come from the collective unconscious and are the basic content of religions, mythologies, legends, and fairytales. They emerge in individuals through dreams and visions.

Association. A spontaneous flow of interconnected thoughts and images around a specific idea, determined by unconscious connections.

Complex. An emotionally charged group of ideas or images. At the "center" of a complex is an archetype or archetypal image.

Constellate. Whenever there is a strong emotional reaction to a person or a situation, a complex has been constellated (activated).

Ego. The central complex in the field of consciousness. A strong ego can relate objectively to activated contents of the unconscious (i.e., other complexes), rather than identifying with them, which appears as a state of possession.

Feeling. One of the four psychic functions. It is a rational function which evaluates the worth of relationships and situations. Feeling must be distinguished from emotion, which is due to an activated complex.

Individuation. The conscious realization of one's unique psychological reality, including both strengths and limitations. It leads to the experience of the Self as the regulating center of the psyche.

Inflation. A state in which one has an unrealistically high or low (negative inflation) sense of identity. It indicates a regression of consciousness into unconsciousness, which typically happens when the ego takes too many unconscious contents upon itself and loses the faculty of discrimination.

Intuition. One of the four psychic functions. It is the irrational function which tells us the possibilities inherent in the present. In contrast to sensation (the function which perceives immediate reality through the physical senses) intuition perceives via the unconscious, e.g., flashes of insight of unknown origin.

115

Participation mystique. A term derived from the anthropologist Lévy-Bruhl, denoting a primitive, psychological connection with objects, or between persons, resulting in a strong unconscious bond.

Persona (Latin, "actor's mask"). One's social role, derived from the expectations of society and early training. A strong ego relates to the outside world through a flexible persona; identification with a specific persona (doctor, scholar, artist, etc.) inhibits psychological development.

Projection. The process whereby an unconscious quality or characteristic of one's own is perceived and reacted to in an outer object or person. Projection of the anima or animus onto a real women or man is experienced as falling in love. Frustrated expectations indicate the need to withdraw projections, in order to relate to the reality of other people.

Puer aeternus (Latin, "eternal youth"). Indicates a certain type of man who remains too long in adolescent psychology, generally associated with a strong unconscious attachment to the mother (actual or symbolic). Positive traits are spontaneity and openness to change. His female counterpart is the **puella,** an "eternal girl" with a corresponding attachment to the father-world.

Self. The archetype of wholeness and the regulating center of the personality. It is experienced as a transpersonal power which transcends the ego, e.g., God.

Senex (Latin, "old man"). Associated with attitudes that come with advancing age. Negatively, this can mean cynicism, rigidity and extreme conservatism; positive traits are responsibility, orderliness and self-discipline. A well-balanced personality functions appropriately within the puer-senex polarity.

Shadow. An unconscious part of the personality characterized by traits and attitudes, whether negative or positive, which the conscious ego tends to reject or ignore. It is personified in dreams by persons of the same sex as the dreamer. Consciously assimilating one's shadow usually results in an increase of energy.

Symbol. The best possible expression for something essentially unknown. Symbolic thinking is non-linear, right-brain oriented; it is complementary to logical, linear, left-brain thinking.

Transcendent function. The reconciling "third" which emerges from the unconscious (in the form of a symbol or a new attitude) after the conflicting opposites have been consciously differentiated, and the tension between them held.

Transference and countertransference. Particular cases of projection, commonly used to describe the unconscious, emotional bonds that arise between two persons in an analytic or therapeutic relationship.

Uroboros. The mythical snake or dragon that eats its own tail. It is a symbol both for individuation as a self-contained, circular process, and for narcissistic self-absorption.

Bibliography

Bart, Pauline. "Depression in Middle-aged Women." *Women in Sexist Society.* Ed. V. Gornick and B.K. Moran. Basic Books, New York, 1971.

Becker, Ernest. *The Denial of Death.* The Free Press (Macmillan), New York, 1973.

Benedek, Therese. "Investigation of the Sexual Cycle in Women." *Archives of General Psychiatry,* 1963.

Black, Kurt. *Transition to Aging and the Self Image.* Duke University, 1971.

Breen, Dana. "The Mother and the Hospital." *Tearing the Veil.* Ed. Susan Lipschitz. Routledge & Kegan Paul, London, 1978.

Campbell, Joseph. *The Hero with a Thousand Faces* (Bollingen Series XVII). Princeton University Press, Princeton, 1973.

———. *The Masks of God.* 4 vols. Penguin Books, New York, 1976.

Carter, Nancy C. "Demeter and Persephone in Margaret Atwood's Novels: Mother-Daughter Transformations." *Journal of Analytical Psychology,* vol. 24, no. 4 (October 1979).

Cooper, Wendy. *No Change.* Arrow Books, New York, 1976.

Corsa, Helen Storm. "Psychoanalytic Concepts of Creativity and Aging." *Journal of Geriatric Psychology,* 1973.

Dempsey, P.J.R. "So That's What It's All About." University College, Cork, 1977.

Deutsch, Helene. *The Psychology of Women,* vol. 2. Grune & Stratton, New York, 1945.

Diagram Group. *Woman's Body: An Owner's Manual.* Corgi, New York, 1978.

Ehrenreich, Barbara, and Deirdre English. *Witches, Midwives and Nurses.* Writers & Readers Publishing Co-operative, London, 1976.

Eliade, Mircea. *Myths, Dreams and Mysteries.* Fontana, London, 1974.

Erikson, Erik. "Womanhood and the Inner Space." *Daedalus Journal of the American Academy of Arts and Sciences,* Spring 1964.

Frazer, J.G. *The Golden Bough.* Macmillan, London, 1957.

Freud, Sigmund. *Outline of Psychoanalysis.* Hogarth Press, London, 1949.

Fried, Barbara. *The Middle Age Crisis.* Harper & Row, New York, 1976.

Glass, R. *Women's Choice: A Guide to Contraception, Fertility, Abortion, and Menopause.* Basic Books, New York, 1982.

Gordon, Rosemary. *Dying and Creating* (Library of Analytical Psychology, vol. 4). Academic Press, London, 1978.

Gornick, V., and B.K. Moran, eds. *Women in Sexist Society.* Basic Books, New York, 1971.

Greene, J.G., and D.J. Cooke. "Life Stress and Symptoms at the Climacterium." *British Journal of Psychiatry,* 1979.

Hannah, Barbara. *Encounters with the Soul: Active Imagination as Developed by C.G. Jung.* Sigo Press, Santa Monica, 1981.

Harding, Esther. *Women's Mysteries, Ancient and Modern.* Rider, London, 1971.

Hauser, Arnold. *Social History of Art.* Routledge & Kegan Paul, London, 1951.

Hubback, Judith. "Reflections on the Psychology of Women." *Journal of Analytical Psychology,* vol. 23, no. 2 (April 1978).

Jung, C.G. *The Collected Works* (Bollingen Series XX). 20 vols. Trans. R.F.C. Hull. Ed. H. Read, M. Fordham, G. Adler, Wm. McGuire. Princeton University Press, Princeton, 1953-1979.

———, and C. Kerényi. *Introduction to a Science of Mythology.* Routledge & Kegan Paul, London, 1951.

Jung, Emma. *Animus and Anima.* Spring Publications, Zurich, 1978.

Keen, Ernest. *A Primer in Phenomenological Psychology.* Holt, Rinehart & Winston, New York, 1975.

King, Pearl. "Notes on the Psychoanalysis of Older Patients." *Journal of Analytical Psychology,* vol. 19, no. 1 (January 1974).

Klaus, Hannah. "The Menopause in Gynaecology." *Journal of Medical Education,* 1974.

Lipschitz, Susan, ed. *Tearing the Veil.* Routledge & Kegan Paul, London, 1978.

Lopez, M.C., et al. *Menopause: A Self Care Manual.* Santa Fe Health Education Project, Santa Fe, 1980.

MacCurtain, Margaret, and Donncha O'Corrain, eds. *Women in Irish Society.* The Women's Press, Dublin, 1978.

Maslow, Abraham. *Toward a Psychology of Being.* Van Nostrand, Princeton, 1962.

Masters and Johnson. *Human Sexual Inadequacy.* Little, Brown & Co., Boston, 1970.

Matriarchy Study Group. *Menstrual Taboos.* London, 1977.

Mead, Margaret. *Male and Female.* Victor Gollancz, London, 1949.

Miller, Jean Baker, ed. *Psychoanalysis and Women.* Penguin Books, London, 1974.

Millette, Brenda, and Joellen Hawkins. *The Passage through Menopause: Women's Lives in Transition.* Reston Publishing Co., Reston, VA, 1983.

Morgan, Elaine. *The Descent of Women.* Souvenir Press, London, 1972.

Neugarten, Bernice. "A New Look at the Menopause." *Psychology Today,* December 1967.

Neumann, Erich. *Amor and Psyche* (Bollingen Series LIV). Trans. R. Manheim. Princeton University Press, Princeton, 1971.

———. *The Great Mother* (Bollingen Series XLVII). Trans. R. Manheim. Princeton University Press, Princeton, 1972.

Perera, Sylvia Brinton. *Descent to the Goddess: A Way of Initiation for Women.* Inner City Books, Toronto, 1981.

Redlich, Patricia. "Women and the Family." *Women in Irish Society.* Ed. Margaret MacCurtain and Donncha O'Corrain. The Women's Press, Dublin, 1978.

Reitz, Rosetta. *Menopause: A Positive Approach.* Penguin Books, New York, 1977.

Robinson, Mary. "Women and the New Irish State." *Women in Irish Society.* Ed. Margaret MacCurtain and Donncha O'Corrain. The Women's Press, Dublin, 1978.

Rose, Catherine. *The Female Experience.* Arlen House, Galway, 1975.

Scharf-Kluger, Rivkah. "Old Testament Roots of Women's Spiritual Problems." *Journal of Analytical Psychology,* vol. 23, no. 2 (April 1978).

Schwartz-Salant, Nathan. *Narcissism and Character Transformation: The Psychology of Narcissistic Character Disorders.* Inner City Books, Toronto, 1982.

Sheehy, Gail. *Pathfinders.* William Morrow & Co., New York, 1981.

Shuttle, Penelope, and Peter Redgrove. *The Wise Wound: Menstruation and Everywoman.* Victor Gollancz, London, 1978.

Singer, June. *Androgyny.* Routledge & Kegan Paul, London, 1977.

Skultans, Vieda. "The Symbolic Significance of Menstruation and the Menopause." *Man,* 1970.

Smallwood, Kathie, and Dorothy Van Dyck. "Menopause Counseling: Coping with Realities and Myths." *Journal of Sex Education Therapy,* 1978.

Studd, John. "Management of the Menopause." London, 1976.

Thompson, Clara. *On Women.* New American Library, New York, 1971.

Van Gennep, Arnold. *The Rites of Passage.* University of Chicago Press, Chicago, 1960.

Verne, Georges. "Individuation and the Emergence of the Unexpected." *Journal of Analytical Psychology,* vol. 14, no. 1 (January 1969).

Weideger, Paula. *Menstruation and Menopause: The Physiology and Psychology: The Myth and the Reality.* Delta Books, New York, 1977.

Weigle, Marta. *Spiders and Spinsters.* University of New Mexico Press, Albuquerque, 1982.

Woodman, Marion. *Addiction to Perfection: The Still Unravished Bride.* Inner City Books, Toronto, 1982.

Index

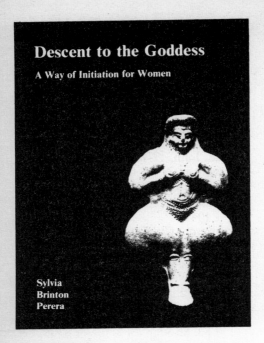

Descent to the Goddess

A Way of Initiation for Women

Sylvia
Brinton
Perera

6. Descent to the Goddess: A Way of Initiation for Women.
Sylvia Brinton Perera (New York). ISBN 0-919123-05-8. 112 pp. $12

A highly original and provocative book about women's freedom and the need for an inner, female authority in a masculine-oriented society.

Combining ancient texts and modern dreams, the author, a practising Jungian analyst, presents a way of feminine initiation. Inanna-Ishtar, Sumerian Goddess of Heaven and Earth, journeys into the underworld to Ereshkigal, her dark "sister," and returns. So modern women must descend from their old role-determined behavior into the depths of their instinct and image patterns, to find anew the Great Goddess and restore her values to modern culture.

Men too will be interested in this book, both for its revelations of women's essential nature and for its implications in terms of their own inner journey.

"The most significant contribution to an understanding of feminine psychology since Esther Harding's *The Way of All Women*."—**Marion Woodman,** Jungian analyst and author of *Addiction to Perfection, The Pregnant Virgin* and *The Owl Was a Baker's Daughter.*

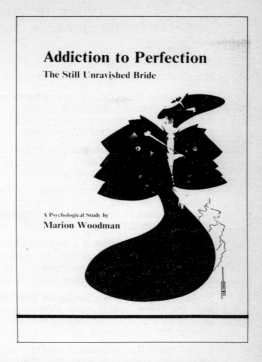

Addiction to Perfection
The Still Unravished Bride

A Psychological Study by
Marion Woodman

12. Addiction to Perfection: The Still Unravished Bride.
Marion Woodman (Toronto). ISBN 0-919123-11-2. 208 pp. $15

"This book is about taking the head off an evil witch." With these words Marion Woodman begins her spiral journey, a powerful and authoritative look at the psychology and attitudes of modern woman.

The witch is a Medusa or a Lady Macbeth, an archetypal pattern functioning autonomously in women, petrifying their spirit and inhibiting their development as free and creatively receptive individuals. Much of this, according to the author, is due to a cultural one-sidedness that favors patriarchal values—productivity, goal orientation, intellectual excellence, spiritual perfection, etc.—at the expense of more earthy, interpersonal values that have traditionally been recognized as the heart of the feminine.

Marion Woodman's first book, *The Owl Was a Baker's Daughter: Obesity, Anorexia Nervosa and the Repressed Feminine,* focused on the psychology of eating disorders and weight disturbances.

Here, with a broader perspective on the same general themes, she continues her remarkable exploration of women's mysteries through case material, dreams, literature and mythology, in food rituals, rape symbolism, Christianity, imagery in the body, sexuality, creativity and relationships.

"It is like finding the loose end in a knotted mass of thread. . . . What a relief! Somebody knows!"—**Elizabeth Strahan,** *Psychological Perspectives.*

Studies in Jungian Psychology
by Jungian Analysts

Limited Edition Paperbacks

Prices and payment in U.S. dollars (except for Canadian orders)

1. The Secret Raven: Conflict and Transformation.
Daryl Sharp (Toronto). ISBN 0-919123-00-7. 128 pp. $13
A practical study of *puer* psychology, including dream interpretation and material on
midlife crisis, the provisional life, the mother complex, anima and shadow. Illustrated.

2. The Psychological Meaning of Redemption Motifs in Fairytales.
Marie-Louise von Franz (Zurich). ISBN 0-919123-01-5. 128 pp. $13
Unique approach to understanding typical dream motifs (bathing, clothes, animals, etc.).

3. On Divination and Synchronicity: The Psychology of Meaningful Chance.
Marie-Louise von Franz (Zurich). ISBN 0-919123-02-3. 128 pp. $13
Penetrating study of irrational methods of divining fate (I Ching, astrology, palmistry, Tarot
cards, etc.), contrasting Western ideas with those of so-called primitives. Illustrated.

**4. The Owl Was a Baker's Daughter: Obesity, Anorexia and the Repressed
Feminine.** Marion Woodman (Toronto). ISBN 0-919123-03-1. 144 pp. $14
A modern classic, with particular attention to the body as mirror of the psyche in weight
disturbances and eating disorders. Based on case studies, dreams and mythology. Illus.

5. Alchemy: An Introduction to the Symbolism and the Psychology.
Marie-Louise von Franz (Zurich). ISBN 0-919123-04-X. 288 pp. $18
Detailed guide to what the alchemists were really looking for: emotional wholeness. Inval-
uable for interpreting images and motifs in modern dreams and drawings. **84 illustrations.**

6. Descent to the Goddess: A Way of Initiation for Women.
Sylvia Brinton Perera (New York). ISBN 0-919123-05-8. 112 pp. $12
A timely and provocative study of the need for an inner, female authority in a masculine-
oriented society. Rich in insights from mythology and the author's analytic practice.

7. The Psyche as Sacrament: C.G. Jung and Paul Tillich.
John P. Dourley (Ottawa). ISBN 0-919123-06-6. 128 pp. $13
Comparative study from a dual perspective (author is Catholic priest and Jungian analyst),
exploring the psychological meaning of religion, God, Christ, the spirit, the Trinity, etc.

8. Border Crossings: Carlos Castaneda's Path of Knowledge.
Donald Lee Williams (Boulder). ISBN 0-919123-07-4. 160 pp. $14
The first thorough psychological examination of the Don Juan novels, bringing Castaneda's
spiritual journey down to earth. Special attention to the psychology of the feminine.

**9. Narcissism and Character Transformation. The Psychology of Narcissistic
Character Disorders.** ISBN 0-919123-08-2. 192 pp. $15
Nathan Schwartz-Salant (New York).
A comprehensive study of narcissistic character disorders, drawing upon a variety of
analytic points of view (Jung, Freud, Kohut, Klein, etc.). Theory and clinical material. Illus.

10. Rape and Ritual: A Psychological Study.
Bradley A. Te Paske (Minneapolis). ISBN 0-919123-09-0. 160 pp. $14
Incisive combination of theory, clinical material and mythology. Illustrated.

11. Alcoholism and Women: The Background and the Psychology.
Jan Bauer (Montreal). ISBN 0-919123-10-4. 144 pp. $14
Sociology, case material, dream analysis and archetypal patterns from mythology.

12. Addiction to Perfection: The Still Unravished Bride.
Marion Woodman (Toronto). ISBN 0-919123-11-2. 208 pp. $15
A powerful and authoritative look at the psychology of modern women. Examines dreams,
mythology, food rituals, body imagery, sexuality and creativity. A continuing best-seller
since its original publication in 1982. Illustrated.

13. Jungian Dream Interpretation: A Handbook of Theory and Practice.
James A. Hall, M.D. (Dallas). ISBN 0-919123-12-0. 128 pp. $13
A practical guide, including common dream motifs and many clinical examples.

14. The Creation of Consciousness: Jung's Myth for Modern Man.
Edward F. Edinger, M.D. (Los Angeles). ISBN 0-919123-13-9. 128 pp. $13
Insightful study of the meaning and purpose of human life. Illustrated.

15. The Analytic Encounter: Transference and Human Relationship.
Mario Jacoby (Zurich). ISBN 0-919123-14-7. 128 pp. $13
Sensitive exploration of the difference between relationships based on projection and
I-Thou relationships characterized by mutual respect and psychological objectivity.

16. Change of Life: Psychological Study of Dreams and the Menopause.
Ann Mankowitz (Santa Fe). ISBN 0-919123-15-5. 128 pp. $13
A moving account of an older woman's Jungian analysis, dramatically revealing the later
years as a time of rebirth, a unique opportunity for psychological development.

17. The Illness That We Are: A Jungian Critique of Christianity.
John P. Dourley (Ottawa). ISBN 0-919123-16-3. 128 pp. $13
Radical study by Catholic priest and analyst, exploring Jung's qualified appreciation of
Christian symbols and ritual, while questioning the masculine ideals of Christianity.

18. Hags and Heroes: A Feminist Approach to Jungian Therapy with Couples.
Polly Young-Eisendrath (Philadelphia). ISBN 0-919123-17-1. 192 pp. $15
Highly original integration of feminist views with the concepts of Jung and Harry Stack
Sullivan. Detailed strategies and techniques, emphasis on feminine authority.

19. Cultural Attitudes in Psychological Perspective.
Joseph Henderson , M.D. (San Francisco). ISBN 0-919123-18-X. 128 pp. $13
Shows how a psychological attitude can give depth to one's world view. Illustrated.

20. The Vertical Labyrinth: Individuation in Jungian Psychology.
Aldo Carotenuto (Rome). ISBN 0-919123-19-8. 144 pp. $14
A guided journey through the world of dreams and psychic reality, illustrating the process
of individual psychological development.

21. The Pregnant Virgin: A Process of Psychological Transformation.
Marion Woodman (Toronto). ISBN 0-919123-20-1. 208 pp. $16
A celebration of the feminine, in both men and women. Explores the wisdom of the body,
eating disorders, relationships, dreams, addictions, etc. Illustrated.

22. Encounter with the Self: William Blake's *Illustrations of the Book of Job.*
Edward F. Edinger, M.D. (Los Angeles). ISBN 0-919123-21-X. 80 pp. $10
Penetrating commentary on the Biblical Job story as a numinous, archetypal event.
Complete with Blake's original 22 engravings.

23. The Scapegoat Complex: Toward a Mythology of Shadow and Guilt.
Sylvia Brinton Perera (New York). ISBN 0-919123-22-8. 128 pp. $13
A hard-hitting study of victim psychology in modern men and women, based on case
material, mythology and archetypal patterns.

24. The Bible and the Psyche: Individuation Symbolism in the Old Testament.
Edward F. Edinger (Los Angeles). ISBN 0-919123-23-6. 176 pp. $15
A major new work relating significant Biblical events to the psychological movement
toward wholeness that takes place in individuals.

25. The Spiral Way: A Woman's Healing Journey.
Aldo Carotenuto (Rome). ISBN 0-919123-24-4. 144 pp. $14
Detailed case history of a fifty-year-old woman's Jungian analysis, with particular attention
to her dreams and the rediscovery of her enthusiasm for life.

26. The Jungian Experience: Analysis and Individuation.
James A. Hall, M.D. (Dallas). ISBN 0-919123-25-2. 176 pp. $15
Comprehensive study of the theory and clinical application of Jungian thought, including
Jung's model, the structure of analysis, where to find an analyst, training centers, etc.

27. Phallos: Sacred Image of the Masculine.
Eugene Monick (Scranton/New York). ISBN 0-919123-26-0. 144 pp. $14
Uncovers the essence of masculinity (as opposed to the patriarchy) through close examination of the physical, mythological and psychological aspects of phallos. **30 illustrations.**

28. The Christian Archetype: A Jungian Commentary on the Life of Christ.
Edward F. Edinger, M.D. (Los Angeles). ISBN 0-919123-27-9. 144 pp. $14
Psychological view of images and events central to the Christian myth, showing their symbolic meaning in terms of personal individuation. **31 illustrations.**

29. Love, Celibacy and the Inner Marriage.
John P. Dourley (Ottawa). ISBN 0-919123-28-7. 128 pp. $13
Shows that without a deeply compassionate relationship to the inner anima/animus, we cannot relate to our intimates or to God, to the full depth of our ability to love.

30. Touching: Body Therapy and Depth Psychology.
Deldon Anne McNeely (Lynchburg, VA). ISBN 0-919123-29-5. 128 pp. $13
Illustrates how these two disciplines, both concerned with restoring life to an ailing human psyche, may be integrated in theory and practice. Focus on the healing power of touch.

31. Personality Types: Jung's Model of Typology.
Daryl Sharp (Toronto). ISBN 0-919123-30-9. 128 pp. $13
Detailed explanation of Jung's model (basis for the widely-used Myers-Briggs Type Indicator), showing its implications for individual development and for relationships. Illus.

32. The Sacred Prostitute: Eternal Aspect of the Feminine.
Nancy Qualls-Corbett (Birmingham). ISBN 0-919123-31-7. 176 pp. $15
Shows how our vitality and capacity for joy depend on rediscovering the ancient connection between spirituality and passionate love. Illustrated. **(Foreword by Marion Woodman.)**

33. When the Spirits Come Back.
Janet O. Dallett (Seal Harbor, WA). ISBN 0-919123-32-5. 160 pp. $14
An analyst examines herself, her profession and the limitations of prevailing attitudes toward mental disturbance. Interweaving her own story with descriptions of those who come to her for help, she details her rediscovery of the integrity of the healing process.

34. The Mother: Archetypal Image in Fairy Tales.
Sibylle Birkhäuser-Oeri (Zurich). ISBN 0-919123-33-3. 176 pp. $15
Compares processes in the unconscious with common images and motifs in folk-lore. Illustrates how positive and negative mother complexes affect us all, with examples from many well-known fairy tales and daily life. **(Edited by Marie-Louise von Franz.)**

35. The Survival Papers: Anatomy of a Midlife Crisis.
Daryl Sharp (Toronto). ISBN 0-919123-34-1. 160 pp. $15
Jung's major concepts—persona, shadow, anima and animus, complexes, projection, typology, active imagination, individuation, etc.—are dramatically presented in the immediate context of an analysand's process. And the analyst's.

36. The Cassandra Complex: Living with Disbelief.
Laurie Layton Schapira (New York). ISBN 0-919123-35-X. 160 pp. $15
Shows how unconscious, prophetic sensibilities can be transformed from a burden into a valuable source of conscious understanding. Includes clinical material and an examination of the role of powerfully intuitive, medial women through history. Illustrated.

37. Dear Gladys: The Survival Papers, Book 2
Daryl Sharp (Toronto). ISBN 0-919123-36-8. 144 pp. $15
An entertaining and instructive continuation of the story begun in *The Survival Papers* (title 35). Part textbook, part novel, part personal exposition.

Prices and payment (check or money order) in $U.S. (in Canada, $Cdn)

Please add $1 per book (bookpost) or $3 per book (airmail)

INNER CITY BOOKS
Box 1271, Station Q, Toronto, Canada M4T 2P4